RESTORE YOUR PRIME

A Comprehensive Physician's Guide to Modern Male Sexual Health, Performance Optimization, and Life-Changing Interventions

GEORGE K. IBRAHIM, M.D., MBA

ISBN 978-1-7346866-5-4

Published by

Platinum Media Solutions
Charlotte, NC

704-200-2239

PlatinumMediaSolutions.com

DEDICATION

To every man who refuses to believe that his best days are behind him.

To my patients, who trusted me with their journey back to vitality.

To my family, who supported my own transformation.

To my staff, who are the World's Best!

And to the countless men who were told to "just accept it" —this book is proof that you don't have to.

Contents

FOREWORD

I'll never forget the conversation that changed everything.

A successful executive sat across from me in my office - fit, intelligent, accomplished by every measure. But his eyes told a different story. He was exhausted. His marriage was struggling. His motivation had evaporated. At 52, he felt as if he were watching his life through a foggy window.

"Doc," he said, "everyone tells me this is just what happens when you get older. But I can't accept that. There has to be another answer."

He was right. There is another answer.

Over my decades practicing medicine, first as a urologist at Duke, then through my training in Anti-Aging and Regenerative Medicine, and now at Biltmore Restorative Medicine, I've seen a disturbing pattern. Men in their 40s, 50s, and 60s are told to accept declining energy, diminishing sexual performance, weight gain, brain fog, and loss of muscle mass as inevitable consequences of aging.

But here's what most doctors won't tell you: These symptoms aren't normal aging. They're signs of hormonal decline that can be measured, understood, and optimized.

When I was diagnosed with multiple sclerosis over ten years ago, I had to retire from surgery. It forced me to reevaluate everything I thought I knew about medicine and aging. That personal journey led me to hormone optimization and regenerative medicine, fields that don't just manage symptoms but actually restore function and vitality.

The difference between traditional medicine and what you'll learn in this book is simple. Traditional medicine asks, "Are your hormone levels dangerous?" I ask, "Are your hormone levels optimal?" Those are two very different questions with vastly different outcomes.

I wrote this book because too many men are suffering needlessly. They're prescribed antidepressants for problems rooted in low testosterone. They're given sleep medications when their hormones disrupt their rest. They're told their erectile dysfunction is "in their head" when it's actually a vascular issue that can be treated.

Restoring Your Prime isn't about turning back the clock; it's about optimizing the biology you have right now. It's about understanding that the fatigue, weight gain, reduced libido, and mental fog you're experiencing aren't character flaws or inevitable decline. They're biochemical imbalances that respond to the right interventions.

In these pages, you'll discover

- Why your testosterone levels matter far more than your doctor probably told you
- How hormone optimization can restore your energy, strength, and sexual vitality
- The truth about "normal" lab ranges versus optimal ranges
- Why bioidentical hormone replacement is different from what you've heard about hormone therapy
- Practical strategies to restore your physical and mental performance

This book challenges the narrative that you should "just accept" diminishing returns as you age. You wouldn't accept a 50% reduction in your business performance, so why take it in your body?

Whether you're 40 and starting to notice changes, or 60 and convinced your best years are gone, this book offers a different path. A path back to feeling like yourself again. A path to restoring your prime.

The executive I mentioned earlier? Six months after optimizing his hormones, he was back in the gym, back in his marriage, and back to feeling like the man he knew he could be. His life didn't just get better; it got great.

That's what I want for you.

Welcome aboard. Let's chart a course back to your prime.

George K. Ibrahim, MD, MBA

Urologist Trained in Anti-Aging and Regenerative Medicine
Biltmore Restorative Medicine & Aesthetics

INTRODUCTION

Your Journey Back to Peak Masculine Vitality

After three decades as a Duke University-trained urologist and oncologist, I've witnessed countless men struggle silently with sexual health challenges that profoundly impact their confidence, relationships, and overall quality of life. My love of medicine and helping others stayed with me throughout my transition from surgeon to hormone optimization specialist, and I've discovered that true sexual wellness extends far beyond what most men understand.

Over ten years ago, I was diagnosed with multiple sclerosis. Rather than put patients at risk, I retired from surgery. During this challenging period, I discovered the transformative power of hormone optimization and regenerative medicine. What I learned changed not only my own life but also led me to open Biltmore Restorative Medicine & Aesthetics in early 2013, with a straightforward goal to be the most highly trained, experienced physician practicing comprehensive sexual wellness and hormone optimization.

THE REALITY OF MODERN MALE SEXUAL HEALTH

Sexual health isn't just about performance; it's about restoring your vitality, confidence, and zest for life. The men who walk into my practice often feel like shadows of their former selves. They're successful in business, devoted to their families, but privately struggling with

- Declining energy and motivation
- Reduced sexual desire and performance
- Loss of muscle mass and increasing body fat
- Mood changes and decreased confidence
- The nagging feeling that their best years are behind them

But here's what I've learned after treating thousands of patients: You don't have to accept decline as inevitable. With the right approach, scientific understanding, and expert guidance, you can feel like YOU again... maybe even better than before.

BEYOND TRADITIONAL MEDICINE

Traditional medicine often treats symptoms in isolation. A urologist might prescribe erectile dysfunction medication. An endocrinologist might focus solely on testosterone numbers. A psychologist might address performance anxiety. But sexual health is a complex interplay of hormonal, physical, psychological, and lifestyle factors that requires a comprehensive, personalized approach.

At Biltmore Restorative Medicine & Aesthetics, we take a holistic approach to patient care. We don't focus on just one specific part of the body or condition; instead, we take a comprehensive approach in our evaluations. Our services are comparable to those offered in larger metropolitan areas, such as Charlotte and Atlanta. In fact, many of our patients consider our services to be superior and fly to us from these cities for treatment.

THE SCIENCE OF RESTORATION

Modern regenerative medicine has revolutionized how we approach male sexual health.

Technologies that were science fiction just a decade ago are now proven, FDA-approved treatments that can

- Restore optimal hormone levels naturally
- Regenerate tissues using your body's own healing factors
- Enhance size and function without surgery
- Improve blood flow and sensation
- Boost confidence and performance

This book represents my commitment to educating men about these possibilities. You'll discover not just what treatments exist, but how they work, who benefits most, and what realistic outcomes look like. Most importantly, you'll understand that you have options... real, scientific options that can transform your life.

YOUR PERSONAL GUIDE TO TRANSFORMATION

Throughout these pages, I'll share insights gained from treating men from their twenties to their eighties, each with unique challenges and goals. You'll learn

- The real science behind hormonal decline and how to address it
- Cutting-edge treatments like the P-Shot®, Priapus Toxin®, and Acoustic Wave therapy
- How lifestyle modifications can amplify medical treatments
- The psychology of sexual confidence and performance
- How to choose the right interventions for your specific situation

WHY PROFESSIONAL GUIDANCE MATTERS

Sexual health optimization isn't something you should attempt alone or with cookie-cutter approaches from franchise clinics. Unlike these commercial operations, independent practices like ours offer

- Physician-led care with decades of specialized experience
- Personalized treatment protocols based on comprehensive evaluation
- Advanced diagnostic testing and ongoing monitoring
- Access to the latest regenerative medicine technologies
- A commitment to your long-term success, not just initial sales

YOUR INVITATION TO RESTORE YOUR PRIME

The journey you're about to embark on isn't just about sexual health; it's about restoring your masculine vitality in all its forms. It's about waking up with energy, approaching challenges with confidence, and feeling genuinely excited about life again.

Whether you're experiencing the first signs of decline or have been struggling for years, the information in this book can change your trajectory. But knowledge alone isn't enough. Fundamental transformation requires action, expert guidance, and a commitment to your own well-being.

As we say at Biltmore Restorative Medicine, we can't wait to help you feel like YOU again!

Your prime years aren't behind you. They're waiting to be restored.

CHAPTER 1

The Modern Crisis in Male Sexual Health: Understanding What's Really Happening

THE SILENT EPIDEMIC AFFECTING MODERN MEN

Almost every man will have a sexual problem at some point in his life, but only a small percentage will share it with their doctors or even their partners. This silence perpetuates what I've come to recognize as a modern epidemic of male sexual dysfunction... one that's affecting younger men at unprecedented rates and preventing them from seeking the available restoration.

In my thirty years of practice, I've witnessed a dramatic shift. Men in their thirties and forties are presenting with symptoms that were once primarily seen in men over sixty. The causes are complex and multifaceted, reflecting the unique challenges of modern life.

But perhaps the most striking moment in my three decades as a urologist came from an unexpected source... a 26-year-old former Marine who walked into my office to assemble equipment we'd purchased.

During lunch, he said something that changed how I practice medicine.

"I overheard some of the questions you were asking patients. I found myself saying 'yes' to many of them."

He'd served three overseas deployments. Young, strong, disciplined. At his hormonal peak, theoretically.

I told him it would be unusual, but we could check.

His testosterone levels came back extremely low.

We started hormone optimization. It changed his life. He went back to school, took the required classes, and sat for the MCATs. Today, he's an orthopedic surgeon.

That moment woke me up to something I'd been missing across 30 years of practice. Even young, strong men can be hormonally deficient. And it's happening at rates I never saw two decades ago.

But understanding this problem required looking beyond conventional thinking. It required recognizing patterns that traditional healthcare often misses, patterns pointing to solutions rooted in restoration rather than resignation.

THE CULTURAL SHIFT NOBODY TALKS ABOUT

When I started my practice, men in their 60s and 70s were stubborn. They wouldn't admit they needed help. Sexual dysfunction was shameful, something to hide.

Today, younger men walk through my door with a completely different mindset.

They've seen commercials for Viagra and Cialis. They know it's acceptable to seek help in this area. They're comfortable talking about sexual wellness in ways their fathers never were.

The cultural barrier is crumbling. However, the medical system has not yet caught up.

Most providers still treat sexual dysfunction as an isolated symptom. They prescribe a pill and send you home.

They're missing the real story your body is trying to tell you.

THE MOST COMMON SEXUAL HEALTH CHALLENGES

During my years at Duke University as a clinical professor of urology, and now in my practice at Biltmore Restorative Medicine, I've identified the most prevalent issues affecting men today

1. Erectile Dysfunction (ED)

Prevalence	Affects 30 million American men
Age Factor	40% of men at age 40, increasing 10% each decade
Modern Reality	Now affecting men in their twenties and thirties at alarming rates

ED isn't just about the inability to achieve an erection. It includes difficulty maintaining erections throughout intercourse, reduced rigidity and firmness, inconsistent performance causing anxiety, and loss of morning erections… often the first warning sign.

The impact extends far beyond the bedroom. Men with ED report decreased self-confidence in all areas of life, relationship strain and communication difficulties, avoidance of intimate situations leading to further relationship deterioration, depression, and anxiety that compounds the original problem, and career impact from reduced confidence and motivation.

2. Low Testosterone Syndrome

This goes far beyond simple numbers on a lab report. Low testosterone affects sexual function (decreased libido, erectile quality, and sexual satisfaction), physical health (muscle loss, fat gain, reduced bone density), mental health (depression, anxiety, cognitive fog, irritability), and energy levels (chronic fatigue, decreased motivation).

The "normal range" myth is particularly dangerous. Most primary care physicians consider testosterone levels "normal" if they fall within a broad range, but this includes the lowest 2.5% of the population. A man with a total testosterone of 322 ng/dL might be told he's "fine" when he's actually in the bottom 5% for optimal male function.

THE HIDDEN EPIDEMIC OF "LOW NORMAL" — AND WHY YOUR LAB REPORT IS LYING TO YOU

Here's something your doctor probably never explained that lab report showing your testosterone is "normal"? It's not telling you what's normal for optimal male health. It's telling you something entirely different, and far less useful.

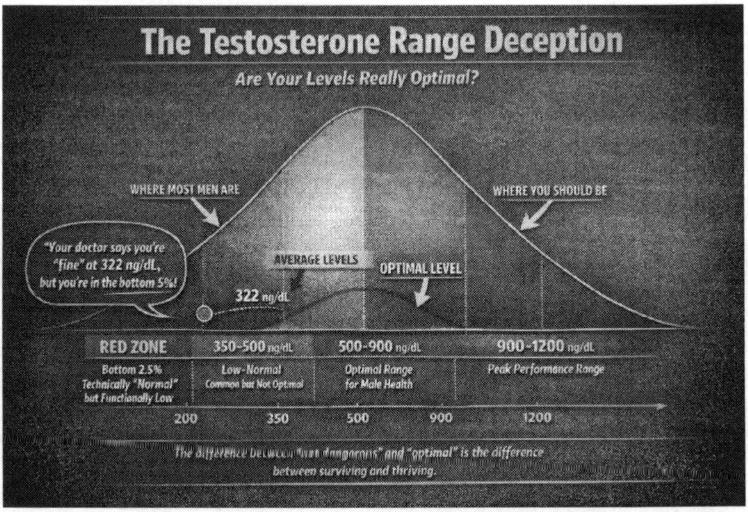

Let me explain.

When you get your testosterone tested, the lab report doesn't show you a "normal range." What it actually shows is something called a "Reference Interval" - two numbers representing the statistical boundaries of what 95% of all tested men fall within. This is calculated using two standard deviations around the mean.

Here's the problem That low number on your report? It's at the 2.5th percentile.

Let that sink in. If your testosterone is at the bottom of the "reference interval," you're in the bottom 2.5% of all men tested. Would you drive your car with only 3% of the oil it needs in the crankcase? Of course not. But your doctor looks at that same 3rd percentile number on your lab report and tells you you're "within normal limits."

This isn't normal. It's a statistical artifact being used as a clinical guideline.

In my practice, I regularly see men whose primary care physicians have dismissed their symptoms because their testosterone falls within this so-called "normal" range. These men typically present with

- Total testosterone levels between 250-400 ng/dL (technically within the reference interval, but functionally inadequate for optimal male performance)
- Symptoms that significantly impact quality of life despite being told they're "fine."
- Years of unsuccessful attempts to address symptoms through other means, such as antidepressants for low mood, sleep medications for fatigue, and relationship counseling for decreased libido

- Relationship problems stemming from reduced sexual drive and emotional flatness
- Professional challenges due to diminished motivation and mental sharpness

The medical establishment has confused "common" with "optimal." Yes, it's common for testosterone to decline with age. Yes, many men have levels in the 200s and 300s. But common doesn't mean normal, and it certainly doesn't mean optimal.

The question isn't "Is your testosterone level dangerous?" The question is "Is your testosterone level optimized for peak male performance?"

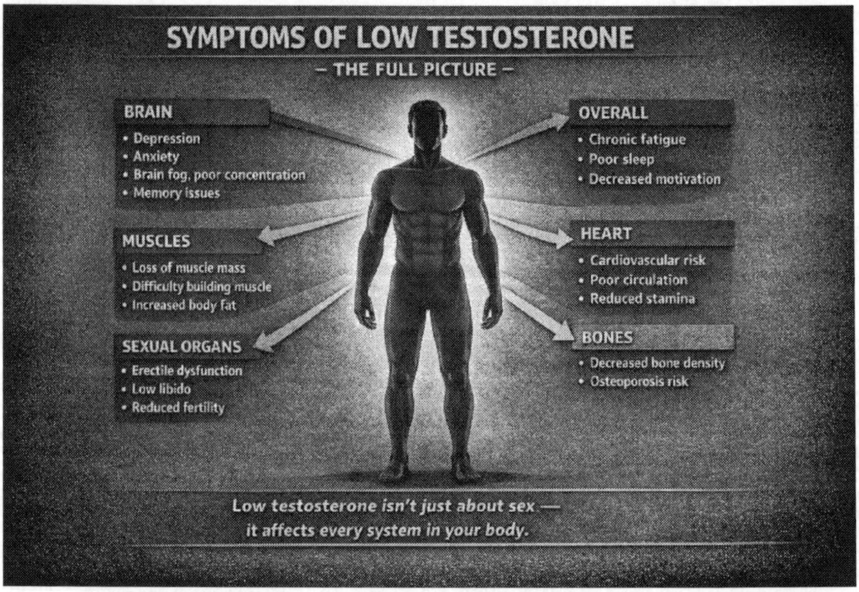

Throughout this book, when I discuss testosterone levels and hormone optimization, I'm not talking about whether you fall somewhere—anywhere—within a reference interval. I'm talking about whether your levels support the energy, strength, mental clarity, and sexual vitality you deserve.

That distinction changes everything.

3. Premature Ejaculation

The most common sexual complaint among men affects 30-40% of men at some point in their lives. It affects men of all ages, though it often begins in early sexual experiences, and involves both psychological and physiological factors.

Premature ejaculation is defined as ejaculation within one minute of penetration (though many men with longer times still feel distressed), lack of control over ejaculation timing, distress or frustration for the man or his partner, and avoidance of sexual activity due to embarrassment.

The condition often creates a vicious cycle. Performance anxiety worsens the condition, avoidance of intimacy strains relationships, reduced sexual confidence affects overall self-esteem, and partner frustration can lead to relationship problems.

4. Performance Anxiety and Psychological Barriers

The mind-body connection in sexual function cannot be overstated. Cultural expectations of masculine performance, relationship stress, communication issues, emotional disconnect, body image concerns, and past trauma from previous negative sexual experiences all play crucial roles.

Performance anxiety often manifests as anticipatory anxiety hours or days before sexual activity, physical symptoms during intimacy (racing heart, sweating, muscle tension), cognitive interference (worried thoughts during sexual activity), and avoidance behaviors that reinforce the anxiety.

One diagnostic question I use regularly reveals this pattern "Do you not have problems with erections when you watch or read pornography, but do have problems with your partner?"

If a man can achieve an erection with porn but not with his partner, he's just told me the problem.

That's a mental issue, not a physical one. It's not something I'm an expert at addressing. That patient needs a therapist, not testosterone. When I identify this pattern, I'm honest. I tell them what I see. I refer them to someone who can help with the psychological component. I stay in my sandbox.

5. Sexual Desire Disorders

Hypoactive sexual desire disorder affects approximately 15% of men. It includes a persistent lack of sexual thoughts or fantasies, an absence of responsive desire to partner's sexual cues, and distress about the lack of sexual interest.

This condition is particularly challenging because partners often take it personally, thinking they're no longer attractive; men feel guilty about not wanting sex as much as they think they should; the problem compounds as relationship tension increases; and treatment requires addressing both individual and relationship factors.

THE DIAGNOSTIC PATHWAY THAT SAVES LIVES

When a man comes to me with erectile dysfunction, I follow a specific pathway that has literally saved lives.

First, check testosterone levels. If they're low, restoration through optimization is the answer.

For younger men planning to have children soon, I use human chorionic gonadotropin. It naturally stimulates the testicles to produce more testosterone, preserving testicular function.

For men not planning children immediately, exogenous bio-identical testosterone is more effective.

But here's what most clinics miss.

If testosterone is optimal and ED persists, that's a warning sign. Something more profound may be happening.

That's when I advise patients to consult their primary care provider to assess cardiovascular risks.

One young man followed this pathway. His testosterone was optimized. ED didn't resolve.

His doctor found a congenital cardiac septal defect. It was decreasing his cardiac output. He underwent cardiac surgery.

His ED resolved completely.

His sexual dysfunction literally saved his life.

This case perfectly illustrates why erectile function is fundamentally a cardiovascular issue... and why treating it superficially can miss life-threatening conditions. The penis serves as a "canary in the coal mine" for cardiovascular health.

The Vascular Connection

Atherosclerosis (plaque buildup that restricts blood flow), endothelial dysfunction (impaired blood vessel function), hypertension (high blood pressure that damages arteries), and diabetes (elevated blood sugar levels that damage nerves and blood vessels) all impact erectile function.

Early Warning System

ED often precedes cardiovascular disease by 3-5 years because the penile arteries are smaller and show damage first. The exact process that affects penile blood flow also affects the coronary arteries. ED can be the first symptom of systemic vascular disease.

What Cookie-Cutter Clinics Would Have Done

Franchise clinics operate on standardized protocols. They're designed for volume, not depth.

In that cardiac case, a cookie-cutter approach would have resulted in one of two outcomes.

- **Option one:** Tell him there was nothing more they could do. Send him home with the problem unsolved.
- **Option two:** Upsell him on intracorporeal injections, penile injections of vasodilators to artificially create erections.

Neither approach would have discovered the heart defect killing him.

This is the fundamental difference between treating symptoms and understanding patients.

Standardized medicine has its place. But sexual dysfunction is rarely standardized.

To understand why sexual dysfunction is becoming more common... and why standard approaches often fail... we need to examine the fundamental changes in modern life affecting male hormonal health.

THE ROOT CAUSES OF MODERN SEXUAL DYSFUNCTION

Hormonal Disruption in the Modern World

Modern life creates a perfect storm for hormonal imbalance through environmental factors and lifestyle choices.

Environmental Factors

Endocrine disruptors in plastics, pesticides, and household chemicals; microplastics in food and water supply; heavy metals and industrial pollutants; and electromagnetic radiation from devices all contribute to hormonal dysfunction.

These environmental toxins are particularly insidious because they accumulate in our bodies over time. Effects may not be immediately apparent but develop gradually; they're virtually impossible to avoid altogether in modern society, and they can affect hormone production at very low concentrations.

Lifestyle Factors

Chronic stress elevates cortisol levels, poor sleep quality disrupts hormone production, sedentary behavior reduces natural testosterone, processed food diets lack essential nutrients, excessive alcohol consumption, and recreational drug use all compound the problem.

WHY THE "WHY" DOESN'T ALWAYS CHANGE TREATMENT

People often ask me about the root causes, such as environmental toxins, chronic stress, and sedentary lifestyles. While these factors absolutely matter for overall health and long-term outcomes, identifying the specific trigger doesn't change the immediate treatment.

Whether testosterone decline stems from a viral illness, chronic stress, environmental factors, or genetic predisposition, the fundamental solution remains the same if testosterone is low, optimization is necessary.

This is why I focus on what I can fix rather than endless investigation into causes. We optimize first. If problems persist, we investigate deeper. This approach enables men to receive the help they need more quickly while also addressing the root causes over time.

The Stress-Hormone-Sexual Function Triangle

Chronic stress creates a cascade of problems through cortisol elevation, which directly suppresses testosterone production, interferes with sleep quality, promotes abdominal fat storage, reduces immune function, and impairs recovery from exercise.

The Vicious Cycle

1. Stress elevates cortisol
2. Cortisol suppresses testosterone
3. Low testosterone reduces stress resilience
4. Reduced resilience increases perceived stress
5. The cycle repeats and intensifies

The Metabolic Connection

Sexual health is closely linked to metabolic health through various pathways.

The Obesity-Sexual Function Connection

Studies show that obese men are significantly more likely to experience erectile dysfunction (up to 3x higher risk), low testosterone (obesity suppresses hormone production), reduced sexual satisfaction for both partners, and decreased fertility (lower sperm count and quality).

The Biochemical Explanation

Aromatase enzyme in fat tissue converts testosterone to estrogen. Insulin resistance interferes with hormone production. Chronic inflammation creates a hostile environment for sexual function. Sleep apnea (common in obesity) further reduces testosterone.

Insulin Resistance and Sexual Function

Poor blood sugar control affects sexual function through nerve damage (diabetic neuropathy affecting sensation), blood vessel damage (reducing blood flow to sexual organs), hormonal disruption (interfering with testosterone production), and increased inflammation (creating systemic health problems).

The Pornography Problem: Creating Unrealistic Expectations

Unfortunately, this is becoming a bigger problem in my practice.

Pornography creates unrealistic expectations. It's not real life. But younger men are growing up thinking it is.

The result is performance anxiety, erectile dysfunction with real partners, and desire disorders that have nothing to do with hormones.

Technology has changed male sexual health in ways we're only beginning to understand.

Pornography-Induced Erectile Dysfunction (PIED) is a growing concern, particularly among younger men. Brain adaptation to artificial stimuli, dopamine dysregulation reducing sensitivity to normal sexual stimuli, conditioning to unrealistic scenarios, and difficulty transitioning to real-world intimacy all contribute to this modern phenomenon.

The Escalation Pattern

Tolerance develops to current material, leading to seeking more extreme content for the same arousal, decreased satisfaction with real partners, and progressive dysfunction with real sexual encounters.

Sedentary Lifestyle Impact

The modern sedentary lifestyle affects sexual health through physical mechanisms, including reduced blood flow (resulting from hours of sitting that compress arteries), muscle atrophy (loss of pelvic floor strength), hormonal changes (decreased testosterone levels due to inactivity), and weight gain (increased body fat, which impacts hormone production).

The Exercise-Testosterone Connection

Resistance training naturally boosts testosterone. Cardiovascular exercise improves blood flow. Regular activity reduces stress and improves mood. Physical fitness enhances body image and confidence.

The Inflammation Factor

Chronic inflammation impacts sexual health through multiple pathways, including endothelial dysfunction (impaired blood vessel function), hormonal disruption (increased cortisol and decreased testosterone), neurological effects (reduced nerve sensitivity and function), and impaired recovery (slower healing after injury or stress).

Sources of Chronic Inflammation

Poor diet (including processed foods and excess sugar), lack of exercise (sedentary lifestyle), chronic stress (elevated cortisol levels), environmental toxins (such as pollution and chemicals), and inadequate sleep (resulting in insufficient recovery time) all contribute.

AGE-RELATED CHANGES: WHAT'S NORMAL VS. WHAT'S TREATABLE

While aging is a natural process, the rate of decline isn't predetermined.

Normal Age-Related Changes

Testosterone levels peak in the low to mid twenties, decreasing by 2-4% annually. By age 50, all men are at about half their peak levels. However, this decline may be accelerated by lifestyle factors and can be significantly slowed or reversed with proper intervention.

Vascular Changes

While aging brings changes like reduced arterial flexibility and decreased nitric oxide production, these aren't inevitable declines. Exercise can improve arterial flexibility. Proper nutrition can enhance nitric oxide production. Treatment can restore compromised blood flow. Even healing and recovery can be optimized. None of these changes is beyond restoration.

The Power of Asking the Right Questions

My comprehensive approach at Biltmore Restorative Medicine starts with something simple: listening.

The patient will nearly always shed light on the problem if the correct questions are asked. And those questions are unique to each patient.

I'm not replacing their primary care provider. When I suspect a systemic cause beyond hormone optimization, I refer them to a specialist.

I stay in my sandbox. But within that sandbox, I dig deep.

Sometimes the problem is purely hormonal. Sometimes it's cardiovascular. Sometimes it's psychological.

This individualized approach reveals patterns that cookie-cutter clinics miss entirely.

WHEN PHYSICAL PROBLEMS CREATE PSYCHOLOGICAL ONES

Sexual dysfunction creates cascading effects. Relationships suffer. Careers take hits, mental health declines.

The good news? Fixing the physical problem usually improves everything.

But not always.

Sometimes there are underlying emotional problems I can't fix. I'm not a counselor. When I suspect emotional issues beyond the physical, I tell patients they should see a therapist.

This is another place where comprehensive care differs from cookie-cutter approaches.

I recognize the limits of what I do. I refer out when needed. The goal isn't to be everything to everyone.

The goal is to get patients the right help at the right time.

THE CASCADE EFFECT: HOW SEXUAL PROBLEMS COMPOUND

Sexual health problems rarely exist in isolation. They create a cascade of issues across multiple domains.

Personal Impact

Reduced self-confidence affecting all areas of life, decreased motivation in work and personal projects, social withdrawal from friends and activities, and depression and anxiety from ongoing frustration all stem from untreated sexual dysfunction.

Relationship Impact

Communication breakdown as couples avoid discussing the problem, emotional distance as physical intimacy decreases, partner blame and resentment on both sides, and relationship dissolution in severe cases create compounding damage.

Professional Impact

Reduced confidence affecting work performance, decreased energy limiting career advancement, increased sick days from related health problems, and lost opportunities due to reduced motivation all demonstrate how sexual health affects every sphere of life.

BREAKING THE SILENCE: CULTURAL BARRIERS TO TREATMENT

Cultural barriers to seeking help unnecessarily perpetuate these problems.

Masculine Stereotypes That Harm

"*Real men don't have sexual problems.*"
This myth prevents men from seeking help.

"*It's just part of getting older.*"
This fatalistic thinking ignores available solutions.

"*I should be able to handle this myself.*"...
This independence can become destructive.

Medical System Limitations

Primary care physicians often lack specialized knowledge in sexual medicine. Fragmented care treats symptoms rather than underlying causes. Limited consultation time prevents a comprehensive evaluation. Overreliance on pharmaceutical solutions ignores root causes.

THE PATH FORWARD: UNDERSTANDING LEADS TO SOLUTIONS

Understanding these challenges is the first step toward restoring your sexual health. The modern epidemic of male sexual dysfunction is real, but it's not inevitable. With the proper knowledge, professional guidance, and commitment to comprehensive wellness, you can overcome these challenges.

The Comprehensive Approach

In my practice at Biltmore Restorative Medicine & Aesthetics, I've seen thousands of men transform their lives through

Medical Interventions

Comprehensive hormonal optimization beyond simple testosterone replacement, advanced regenerative treatments using your body's own healing factors, cutting-edge enhancement procedures for both function and confidence, and precision diagnostic testing to identify all contributing factors.

Lifestyle Modifications

Targeted nutrition programs to support hormone production, exercise protocols specifically designed for sexual health, stress management techniques to break the stress-hormone cycle, and sleep optimization to maximize natural hormone production.

Psychological Support

Performance anxiety treatment using proven techniques, relationship counseling to improve communication and intimacy, body image work to enhance confidence and self-perception, and mindfulness training to improve present-moment awareness.

WHY COOKIE-CUTTER SOLUTIONS DON'T WORK

The key is understanding that sexual health is a complex system requiring a sophisticated, personalized approach focused on restoring your body's natural function. Cookie-cutter solutions from franchise clinics don't work for most men because:

Individual Complexity

Every man's situation is unique, with different contributing factors. Hormone levels vary widely even within "normal" ranges. Psychological factors vary with personality and experience. Relationship dynamics require individualized approaches.

Treatment Interactions

Multiple treatments often work synergistically when properly combined. The timing of interventions can significantly affect outcomes. Dosing and protocols must be adjusted based on individual response. Ongoing monitoring is essential for optimal results.

The Franchise Clinic Problem

Many men turn to franchise "men's clinics" that promise quick fixes but often deliver cookie-cutter protocols that overlook individual differences, prioritize sales-focused approaches over medical care, offer limited diagnostic testing, omit crucial factors, employ inexperienced providers without specialized training, and provide no long-term support after initial treatment.

THE BILTMORE RESTORATIVE MEDICINE DIFFERENCE

As an independent practice with a urologist who has 30+ years of experience, we offer restorative care that goes beyond symptom management.

Expert Medical Care

Comprehensive evaluation addressing all potential factors, advanced diagnostic testing including detailed hormone panels, personalized treatment protocols designed for your unique situation, and ongoing monitoring and adjustment to optimize results.

Cutting-Edge Treatments

P-Shot® (Priapus Shot) using your own growth factors for natural restoration, acoustic wave therapy to improve blood flow naturally, Priapus Toxin® for enhanced appearance and function, RestoreMore girth enhancement using advanced techniques, and precision hormone optimization going beyond basic testosterone.

Comprehensive Support

Long-term relationships focused on your continued success, education, and counseling to help you understand your condition, lifestyle optimization to enhance treatment effectiveness, and partner support when appropriate to improve relationships.

WHAT GIVES ME HOPE AFTER THREE DECADES

I've watched the entire landscape of male sexual health transform.

Thirty years ago, men suffered in silence. They believed sexual dysfunction was inevitable with age. They were too ashamed to seek help.

Today, younger men understand that restoration is possible when problems have causes beyond their control.

They know finding a knowledgeable provider can improve their life. Sometimes it can save their life.

That 26-year-old Marine is now an orthopedic surgeon. The young man with the cardiac septum is alive because his ED led to the discovery of a fatal heart defect.

These aren't isolated cases. They're examples of what happens when we treat sexual health as a window into overall health.

We have the best opportunity for positive results when we ask the right questions, optimize first and investigate more deeply, and refuse to accept cookie-cutter answers to complex problems.

THE MESSAGE FOR MEN STILL SUFFERING IN SILENCE

I stress this to every patient who walks through my door.

There is no shame in seeking help.

If anything, you're doing your relationship a service by addressing the problem. You're choosing restoration over resignation, taking control of your health instead of accepting decline.

I want men to know that if they give us feedback on our interventions, we can adjust treatment. We can refer them to other experts when the problem extends beyond hormone insufficiency.

Sexual dysfunction isn't a character flaw. It's not inevitable aging. It's not something to hide. It's a medical condition with proven solutions.

Sometimes, those solutions are as simple as hormone optimization. Sometimes they reveal deeper health issues that need attention.

Either way, the answer starts with walking through the door.

The Reality Check: Taking Action

Your sexual health challenges aren't a reflection of your worth as a man... they're medical conditions with proven solutions. The question isn't whether help is available, but whether you're ready to take the first step toward restoring your vitality.

The Cost of Waiting

Problems typically worsen over time without intervention. Relationship damage can become irreversible. Erosion of self-confidence affects all areas of life. Health complications from untreated hormonal imbalances multiply.

The Benefit of Action

Proven treatments are available right now. Technology continues to improve with new options emerging. Earlier intervention typically produces better results. Quality-of-life improvements extend far beyond sexual function.

As I tell every patient, "We can restore what's been lost. You can feel like YOU again."

The modern crisis in male sexual health is real, but so are the solutions. The choice is yours: continue accepting it, regard it as inevitable, or take action to restore your masculine vitality and confidence. The question isn't whether help exists. It's whether you're ready to seek it out.

Because on the other side of that decision is a life where you feel like yourself again. Where relationships improve. Where the cascading effects reverse. Where sexual health becomes what it should be, a reflection of overall vitality, not a source of shame.

The silent epidemic is real. But silence doesn't have to be your response.

At Biltmore Restorative Medicine & Aesthetics, we're here to help you make that choice and support you every step of the way toward restored health and renewed vitality.

References

Harman SM, Metter EJ, Tobin JD, et al.
Longitudinal effects of aging on serum total and free testosterone levels in healthy men.
Baltimore Longitudinal Study of Aging.
J Clin Endocrinol Metab. 2001;86(2)724-731. PMID 11158037
https//pubmed.ncbi.nlm.nih.gov/11158037/

Feldman HA, Longcope C, Derby CA, et al.
Age trends in the level of serum testosterone and other hormones in middle-aged men longitudinal results from the Massachusetts male aging study.
J Clin Endocrinol Metab. 2002;87(2)589-598. PMID 11836290
https//pubmed.ncbi.nlm.nih.gov/11836290/

Dos Santos MR, Bhasin S.
Benefits and Risks of Testosterone Treatment in Men with Age-Related Decline in Testosterone.
Annu Rev Med. 2021;7275-91. PMID 33217248
https//pubmed.ncbi.nlm.nih.gov/33217248/

Travison TG, Shackelton R, Araujo AB, et al.
The relative contributions of aging, health, and lifestyle factors to serum testosterone decline in men.
J Clin Endocrinol Metab. 2007;92(2)549-555.PMID 17148559
https//pubmed.ncbi.nlm.nih.gov/17148559/

CHAPTER 2

The Science of Hormonal Decline – How Your Body Changes and Why It Matters

THE HORMONAL SYMPHONY OF MASCULINE VITALITY

Think of your hormonal system as an orchestra. When all instruments play in harmony, you experience optimal health, energy, and sexual function. But when key players start falling out of tune... particularly testosterone... the entire performance suffers. After thirty years of treating men, I've learned that understanding this hormonal symphony is crucial to restoring your vitality.

The complexity of the male hormonal system often surprises my patients. They come in thinking testosterone is the only hormone that matters, but the reality is far more intricate. Your body produces dozens of hormones that work together in carefully orchestrated patterns. When one falls out of balance, it creates a domino effect that can impact everything from your energy levels to your sexual function to your mental clarity.

Let me show you what happens when this hormonal symphony falls out of tune, and, more importantly, how we can restore the harmony.

YOUR TESTOSTERONE IS NORMAL, BUT YOU FEEL TERRIBLE

Let me paint you a picture I see every week in my practice.

The lab report shows a number within the reference range. Your doctor says you're fine.

But you're not fine.

You're gaining weight despite eating less. Your libido has disappeared. You can't build muscle as easily as you used to. Your thinking feels foggy. You're exhausted by 2 pm.

And yet, medically speaking, you're "normal."

Here's what that really means.

The 2.5% Trap

Lab reports display a "Reference Interval" alongside your testosterone results. This range encompasses two standard deviations around the average, meaning that 95% of all tested men fall within it.

That leaves only 2.5% below the low end and 2.5% above the high end.

Your testosterone isn't flagged as "low" until you're at or below the 2.4th percentile. You have to be in the bottom 2.5% of all men tested before the medical system acknowledges a problem.

That's nuts.

If your testosterone is anywhere near the lower end of that vast range, it's low for you. The report doesn't say "normal." It provides a number within a range that spans from barely functional to optimal.

I see men every week whose testosterone sits at the 10th or 15th percentile. Technically "within range." Functionally struggling.

This is one of the most frustrating aspects of my practice. I regularly see men whose primary care physicians have dismissed their symptoms because their testosterone levels technically fall within the "normal" range.

The Problem with Reference Ranges

- Based on diseased populations
- Include men with chronic illnesses
- Age-adjusted: Compare you to other men your age, not optimal levels
- Too broad. Include the bottom 2.5% of the population as "normal."
- Ignore symptoms. Focus on numbers rather than how you feel.

Real Patient Example

John, a 45-year-old executive, came to me after his primary care doctor told him his testosterone level of 311 ng/dL was "fine." He was experiencing chronic fatigue despite adequate sleep, decreased muscle mass despite regular exercise, reduced sexual desire, straining his marriage, mood changes affecting his work performance, and cognitive fog, making decision-making difficult.

While technically "normal," his testosterone was in the bottom 5% of men his age. After optimization to 750 ng/dL, he reported feeling like himself again.

WHAT YOUR BODY IS ACTUALLY TELLING YOU

When a man comes to my practice with low libido, erectile difficulties, trouble gaining muscle, foggy thinking, and weight gain, I'm not looking at his lab report first.

I'm looking at him.

These symptoms are your body's way of screaming that something is wrong. They're not in your head. They're not just aging. They're the direct result of suboptimal testosterone levels.

But here's what I tell men who other physicians have dismissed: You were at your peak testosterone level in your twenties. By age 50, you're at half that peak. By 60, you're at a third. By 70, you're at a quarter.

Yes, you can drive a car with tires that are only half inflated, but it won't perform optimally. The same principle applies to a man trying to function at 60 with half the hormonal resources he had at 25.

Laboratory reference ranges include the lowest 2.5% of the population, meaning a man could have the testosterone level of a 90-year-old and still be told he's "within normal range." But "normal" isn't the same as "optimal."

TESTOSTERONE: THE MASTER CONDUCTOR

Testosterone isn't just about sex drive and muscle mass. It is the master hormone that orchestrates masculine health across multiple systems.

Primary Functions of Testosterone

Sexual Health

Testosterone drives sexual desire and interest, is essential for achieving and maintaining erections, critical for fertility and reproductive health, affects both performance and pleasure, and maintains healthy penile and testicular tissue.

Physical Development

It promotes protein synthesis and muscle growth, prevents osteoporosis and fractures, helps maintain healthy body composition, stimulates healthy blood formation, and maintains masculine physical characteristics.

Cognitive Function

Testosterone improves both short-term and long-term memory, enhances focus and mental clarity, supports confident, decisive thinking, is essential for navigation and problem-solving, and affects how quickly you think and react.

Emotional Regulation

It helps prevent depression and anxiety, supports self-assurance and assertiveness, drives ambition and goal-oriented behavior, helps you cope with life's challenges, and affects how you process and express feelings.

Metabolic Health

Testosterone helps maintain healthy blood sugar levels, supports cellular energy metabolism, supports a healthy lipid profile, supports cardiovascular health, and helps reduce chronic inflammation.

THE TESTOSTERONE PRODUCTION PROCESS

Understanding how testosterone is produced helps explain why so many things can go wrong and why a comprehensive approach to treatment is necessary.

Step 1 Hypothalamic Initiation

The hypothalamus, a small region in your brain, initiates the process by releasing GnRH (Gonadotropin-Releasing Hormone). This happens in pulses throughout the day, with the pattern being crucial for optimal hormone production.

Factors Affecting Hypothalamic Function

Sleep quality (deep sleep is when most GnRH is released), stress levels (chronic stress disrupts normal pulsing patterns), nutrition (adequate calories and nutrients are essential), body fat (both too much and too little fat can disrupt signaling), and age (natural decline in hypothalamic sensitivity over time) all play critical roles.

Step 2 Pituitary Response

The pituitary gland responds to GnRH by releasing two crucial hormones LH (Luteinizing Hormone), which signals the testicles to produce testosterone, and FSH (Follicle-Stimulating Hormone), which stimulates sperm production.

Step 3 Testicular Production

The testicles receive the LH signal and produce testosterone in specialized cells called Leydig cells. This is where hormones are actually synthesized.

Step 4 Conversion and Transport

Once produced, testosterone travels through the bloodstream and can be converted into other essential hormones, DHT (Dihydrotestosterone), a more potent form of testosterone; Estradiol (yes, men need some estrogen for optimal health); and various metabolites, each with specific functions in the body.

This delicate cascade can be disrupted at any point, leading to symptoms that dramatically impact quality of life. That's why comprehensive testing and individualized treatment are essential.

Understanding these production mechanisms is essential because it reveals where things can go wrong... and how we can intervene to restore optimal function.

THE NATURAL DECLINE: WHAT'S NORMAL VS. WHAT'S OPTIMAL

Age-Related Testosterone Changes

Peak Production (Ages 20-25)

Total testosterone typically ranges from 800 to 1200 ng/dL, and free testosterone usually ranges from 15 to 25 ng/dL. This is when men experience peak sexual function, characterized by maximum libido and performance, optimal physical condition, including the best muscle mass and energy, and sharpest cognitive function.

Early Decline (Ages 30-40)

A gradual decrease of 2-4% per year begins, accompanied by subtle symptoms that may not be immediately noticeable. There's a variable response; some men are more affected than others, and lifestyle factors, such as poor habits, accelerate decline.

Noticeable Impact (Ages 40-50)

Significant reduction of 30-50% below peak levels occurs, with obvious symptoms affecting energy, libido, and performance. Body composition changes, including muscle loss and fat gain, become apparent, and mood changes, such as increased irritability and decreased motivation, emerge.

Marked Decline (Ages 50+)

Substantial reduction, often 50% below peak, leads to major symptoms with significant impact on quality of life, health risks, including increased cardiovascular and metabolic problems, and relationship impact through sexual and emotional difficulties.

The Younger Men Problem

Something has changed in the last decade. Younger men are showing up with surprisingly low testosterone levels... men in their 30s and 40s with numbers I'd expect to see in men twenty years older.

The reasons are varied... environmental toxins, processed foods, chronic stress, sleep disorders, and obesity all contribute. But here's the pragmatic truth: the reason doesn't change the management.

Yes, I identify these lifestyle factors in patients, and they need to address them for overall health. Fixing diet, reducing toxin exposure, managing stress... these things matter.

However, most people won't or can't change everything that affects them. That's where bioidentical hormone optimization comes in.

We've Outlived Our Biological Design

Hormone optimization isn't a band-aid. It's not fighting nature.

It's adapting to the fact that we've already beaten nature by living decades beyond our biological design.

Consider this evolutionary perspective.

Cave men died in their mid-thirties. Now we live to 100. Few mammals live past their reproductive age. While men can theoretically father a child at 60, that's not what our gonads were designed for.

Incidentally, human women, elephants, some toothed whales, and some chimpanzees are the only mammals that live past their reproductive age. A woman's ovaries fizzle out around the age of 50, when they enter menopause.

Our hormonal systems were designed for a lifespan of approximately 35 years, possibly 40.

We're asking them to function optimally for 80 or 90 years. That's not reasonable without intervention.

This reframe is significant because it alters your perspective on treatment. You're not trying to be superhuman. You're trying to maintain function in a body that's operating well beyond its evolutionary warranty.

SYMPTOMS OF SUBOPTIMAL TESTOSTERONE

Physical Symptoms

Chronic fatigue not improved by rest, decreased muscle mass despite exercise, increased body fat, particularly around the midsection, reduced strength and exercise capacity, joint aches and stiffness, and hot flashes or temperature regulation problems all indicate suboptimal testosterone.

Sexual Symptoms

Decreased libido or sexual interest, erectile dysfunction or reduced firmness, reduced sexual satisfaction for both partners, fewer spontaneous erections (especially morning erections), and reduced genital sensitivity are common manifestations.

Cognitive Symptoms

Brain fog or mental cloudiness, poor concentration and focus, memory problems, both short and long-term, reduced mental energy, and difficulty with complex tasks signal a hormonal imbalance.

Emotional Symptoms

Irritability and mood swings, depression or persistent sadness, anxiety and worry, reduced motivation and drive, and social withdrawal often accompany low testosterone.

COMPREHENSIVE HORMONE TESTING BEYOND BASIC TESTOSTERONE

At Biltmore Restorative Medicine, we perform the most comprehensive hormone evaluation available. Most doctors order a simple "total testosterone" test, but this tells only a small part of the story.

Beyond Total Testosterone

Most clinics check total testosterone and call it a day. That's like checking your bank account balance without knowing how much of it you can actually spend.

At Biltmore Restorative Medicine, we look beyond total testosterone. We examine free testosterone, the hormone that's not bound and therefore available to work in your body.

We check SHBG to see if it's high, which would bind up your testosterone and make it unavailable. We measure estrogen levels because some men convert too much testosterone to estrogen, which creates its own problems. We examine FSH and LH to determine whether a pituitary issue is affecting hormone production.

This comprehensive testing reveals what's actually happening in your hormonal system, not just a single number on a spectrum.

ESSENTIAL HORMONE MARKERS

Testosterone Panel

Total Testosterone	Overall hormone production
Free Testosterone	The biologically active hormone not bound to proteins

Bioavailable Testosterone Hormone	Available for use by tissues
SHBG (Sex Hormone-Binding Globulin)	A Protein that binds and transports hormones

Understanding these relationships is crucial. A man might have normal total testosterone but high SHBG, meaning very little free testosterone is available for use. This is why symptoms can persist despite "normal" lab values.

Supporting Hormone Analysis

Estradiol (E2)	Men need some estrogen, but too much can cause problems
DHT (Dihydrotestosterone)	The most potent form of testosterone, but DHT can cause issues such as acne and hair loss
LH and FSH	Indicate whether the problem is testicular or pituitary
Prolactin	Elevated levels can suppress testosterone production

The Estrogen Conversion Problem

Here's something that surprises most men you need some estrogen for memory and bone health.

But too much estrogen leads to man boobs, belly fat, decreased libido, and erectile problems.

Some men convert testosterone to estrogen at higher rates than others. It's individualized. We monitor for this and treat the men who convert too much.

I had a patient, 60 years old, with a fantastic testosterone level of 910. Most doctors would see that number and assume he's fine. However, his estrogen levels were higher than those of most women.

He had severe erectile problems despite the high testosterone. Just treating his conversion problem fixed everything. We didn't need to add testosterone at all.

A standardized, "recipe" approach would have missed this entirely. He would have gotten more testosterone, which would have converted to even more estrogen, making his problems worse.

SUPPORTING HORMONE SYSTEMS

Thyroid Function

Many men with sexual health issues have undiagnosed thyroid problems. We test TSH (a pituitary hormone that stimulates the thyroid), Free T4 (the storage form of thyroid hormone), Free T3 (the active form of thyroid hormone), Reverse T3 (an inactive form that can interfere with thyroid function), and thyroid antibodies to check for autoimmune thyroid disease.

Adrenal Function

Chronic stress can devastate hormone production. We assess cortisol (the primary stress hormone that should be high in the morning and low at night), DHEA-S (a precursor hormone that declines with age and stress), the cortisol/DHEA ratio (which indicates stress resilience), and the 24-hour cortisol pattern to determine whether your stress response is healthy.

Growth Hormone System

Necessary for recovery and vitality, we test IGF-1 (which indicates growth hormone production) and perform growth hormone stimulation tests when indicated. We also assess sleep quality, as most growth hormone is produced during deep sleep.

Metabolic Markers

Essential for overall health are insulin and glucose (check for diabetes and insulin resistance), Hemoglobin A1c (average blood sugar over 3 months), a lipid panel (cholesterol and triglycerides), and inflammatory markers such as C-reactive protein and ESR.

ADVANCED DIAGNOSTIC MARKERS

Comprehensive Metabolic Assessment

Complete Blood Count (CBC) to check for anemia or blood disorders, Comprehensive Metabolic Panel (CMP) for liver and kidney function, prostate health markers including PSA and free PSA for safety monitoring, and nutritional status including B12, vitamin D, folate, zinc, and magnesium.

Specialized Testing When Indicated

Sleep study if sleep apnea is suspected; cardiac evaluation for men with cardiovascular risk factors; genetic testing for specific hormone-related conditions; and heavy metal testing if environmental exposure is suspected.

THE DOMINO EFFECT OF HORMONAL IMBALANCE

When testosterone levels decline, it triggers a cascade of negative changes throughout your body. Understanding this domino effect helps explain why hormone optimization can have such dramatic benefits.

Sexual Function Deterioration

Primary Sexual Impact

Reduced libido (loss of sexual thoughts, fantasies, and interest), erectile dysfunction (difficulty achieving or maintaining erections), decreased sensitivity (reduced pleasure and sensation during sexual activity), performance anxiety (psychological impact of physical changes), and relationship strain (impact on partner and relationship dynamics) all emerge.

The Vicious Cycle Sexual problems create stress, which elevates cortisol, which further suppresses testosterone, making the sexual problems worse. This cycle can quickly spiral out of control without intervention.

Physical Changes

Muscle Loss (Sarcopenia)

The rate of decline averages 3-8% loss of muscle mass per decade after age 30, with strength reduction disproportionate to size loss. This creates a metabolic impact, as muscle tissue burns calories even at rest, leading to functional decline, making daily activities difficult, and increasing the risk of injury due to weaker muscles and bones.

Body Composition Changes

Fat accumulation, particularly around the midsection (visceral fat), results in a gradual shift toward a higher body fat percentage in the muscle-to-fat ratio. Additionally, bone density loss increases the risk of osteoporosis and fractures, while skin changes, stemming from reduced collagen production, affect appearance.

Metabolic Disruption

Insulin Resistance

Low testosterone contributes to difficulty processing blood sugar through cellular resistance (cells become less responsive to insulin), increased diabetes risk with Type 2 diabetes development, weight gain, particularly with abdominal fat storage, and energy crashes from blood sugar swings affecting energy.

Cardiovascular Impact

Cholesterol changes with increased LDL and decreased HDL; a tendency toward hypertension; reduced flexibility; and increased plaque formation in arterial health all follow.

Psychological Impact

Mood and Cognitive Changes

Clinical depression rates are higher in men with low testosterone, along with increased anxiety, worry, and nervousness, irritability with short temper and emotional volatility, cognitive decline, including memory problems and reduced mental clarity, and motivation loss with decreased drive and ambition.

Social and Professional Impact

Reduced confidence affecting work and personal relationships, social withdrawal with less interest in activities and friendships, performance decline with reduced effectiveness at work, and relationship problems straining marriage and family relationships compound the difficulties.

To understand why hormone decline has accelerated in recent generations, it is necessary to examine the environmental and lifestyle factors specific to modern life.

MODERN LIFESTYLE FACTORS ACCELERATING DECLINE

While aging is a natural process, modern life significantly accelerates the decline in hormone levels. Understanding these factors helps explain why men today experience symptoms earlier and more severely than previous generations.

Environmental Toxins: The Hidden Threat

Endocrine Disruptors

These chemicals interfere with hormone production and function.

Bisphenol A (BPA)

Found in plastic bottles, canned food linings, and receipts, BPA mimics estrogen and suppresses testosterone. Exposure is virtually unavoidable in modern life and accumulates in tissues over time.

Phthalates

Found in personal care products, plastics, and fragrances, phthalates reduce testosterone production through skin absorption, inhalation, and ingestion. Higher exposure is particularly concerning as it's linked to fertility problems.

Pesticides and Herbicides

Atrazine (a common herbicide that affects hormone production), organophosphates (pesticides that disrupt endocrine function), and glyphosate (a widely used herbicide with potential hormone effects) create cumulative exposure, with effects that build over a lifetime.

Heavy Metals

Lead (stored in bones and released during times of stress), mercury (particularly from eating large fish), cadmium (from cigarette smoke and industrial pollution), and aluminum (from antiperspirants and cookware) all contribute.

DIETARY FACTORS: FOOD AS MEDICINE OR POISON

Testosterone-Lowering Foods

Processed Foods contain trans fats that directly suppress testosterone production; high sodium contributes to inflammation and blood pressure issues; preservatives have endocrine-disrupting properties; and artificial additives have unknown long-term effects on hormones.

Sugar and Refined Carbohydrates cause insulin spikes that repeatedly suppress testosterone, create inflammation, leading to chronic inflammatory states, promote weight gain, particularly in abdominal fat, which produces estrogen, and cause energy crashes, leading to stress and cortisol elevation.

Excessive Alcohol directly inhibits testosterone production, disrupts sleep, interferes with overnight hormone production, stresses the liver, impairs hormone metabolism, and depletes vitamins and minerals needed for hormone production.

Soy Products (Controversial) contain phytoestrogens (plant compounds that may mimic estrogen), although individual variation means that some men are more sensitive to them than others. Processing matters, as fermented soy may be less problematic, and dosage is dependent... moderate consumption is likely not harmful.

Nutritional Deficiencies

Critical Nutrients for Hormone Production

Zinc is an essential cofactor in the synthesis of testosterone. Deficiency signs include reduced testosterone and poor wound healing. Sources include oysters, red meat, and pumpkin seeds. Supplementation with 15-30mg daily is adequate for most men.

Vitamin D is actually a hormone precursor, not a vitamin. Most men have suboptimal levels in what amounts to a deficiency epidemic. Testing should aim for blood levels of 40-60 ng/mL. Sources include sun exposure, fatty fish, and supplementation.

Magnesium is required for over 300 enzymatic reactions and is rapidly depleted during times of stress. It's essential for high-quality, restorative sleep. Magnesium glycinate is the best absorbed form.

Omega-3 Fatty Acids reduce inflammation and support hormone production. Most diets are severely lacking, creating modern deficiencies. The ratio matters... omega-6 to omega-3 should be 41 or less. Sources include wild-caught fish and algae supplements.

CHRONIC STRESS: THE HORMONE KILLER

Chronic stress creates a hormonal environment hostile to testosterone production.

The Stress-Hormone Connection

Cortisol Elevation directly inhibits testosterone production. The body prioritizes stress response over reproduction through resource competition. Modern stress rarely resolves, leading to chronic activation. High cortisol levels interfere with sleep quality, further exacerbating the problem.

The Modern Stress Epidemic

Work stress encompasses financial pressure from job security and economic uncertainty, performance demands that constantly put pressure to achieve, technology that keeps us continually connected and never truly off, and commuting, which creates daily stress from traffic and travel.

Relationship Stress involves communication problems as modern relationships become more complex, financial strain due to money problems affecting couples, parenting pressure with an intense focus on child achievement, and social media that creates constant comparisons with others.

Information Overload creates news anxiety from constant exposure to negative news, decision fatigue from too many choices in modern life, FOMO (fear of missing out), constant anxiety, and digital addiction, causing dopamine dysregulation from devices.

SLEEP DISORDERS WHEN RECOVERY BECOMES IMPOSSIBLE

Quality sleep is when your body produces the most testosterone. Modern life systematically destroys sleep quality.

Sleep and Hormone Production

Natural Rhythm

During deep sleep, most testosterone is produced. REM sleep is essential for psychological recovery. Growth hormone is also produced during deep sleep. Sleep allows cortisol levels to normalize and reset.

Modern Sleep Disruptors

Sleep Apnea affects 25% of men over 40. Its severity can reduce testosterone by 50% or more. The condition often goes undiagnosed for years. CPAP therapy can restore normal hormone production.

Blue Light Exposure suppresses melatonin production through its mechanism. Sources include phones, tablets, computers, and LED lights. Timing is particularly problematic in evening hours. Solutions include blue light-blocking glasses and red light in the evening.

Caffeine and Stimulants have a half-life of 6-8 hours in your system. Even if you fall asleep, your sleep quality is reduced. Timing recommendations suggest no caffeine after 2 PM for most people. Dependency creates a cycle of poor sleep and increased caffeine need.

THE OBESITY-HORMONE CONNECTION A VICIOUS CYCLE

Excess body fat, particularly abdominal fat, creates a vicious cycle that's particularly damaging to hormone production.

How Obesity Lowers Testosterone

The aromatase enzyme is concentrated in fat tissue, particularly in abdominal fat. Its function is to convert testosterone to estrogen. More fat tissue equals more aromatase, which equals less testosterone. This creates a vicious cycle where lower testosterone makes it harder to lose fat.

Insulin Resistance develops as fat tissue becomes resistant to insulin. This effect impairs hormone production and regulation. Fat tissue produces inflammatory compounds, which in turn create inflammation. Obesity often leads to sleep apnea, further compounding sleep breathing problems.

How Low Testosterone Promotes Obesity

Metabolic Slowdown occurs through muscle loss, which reduces muscle mass and lowers metabolic rate. Decreased energy reduces motivation for physical activity. Low testosterone worsens insulin sensitivity. The body prefers to store rather than burn fat.

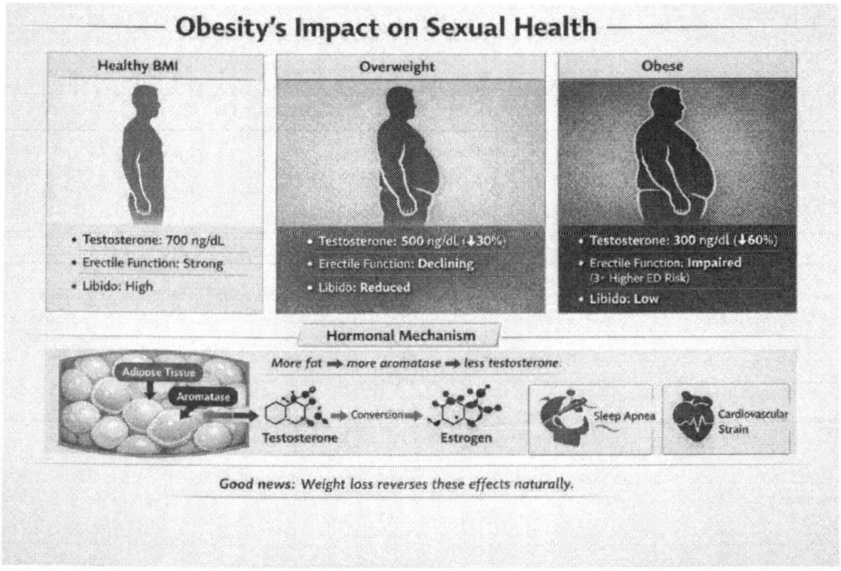

THE CARDIOVASCULAR-HORMONE CONNECTION

Your cardiovascular health and hormone levels are closely linked, forming another vital feedback loop.

How Low Testosterone Affects Heart Health

Lipid Changes

LDL cholesterol tends to increase in individuals with low testosterone levels. HDL cholesterol levels often decrease when testosterone levels are low. Triglycerides may increase, especially in individuals with insulin resistance. LDL particles may become smaller and more dangerous.

Vascular Function

Testosterone supports healthy blood vessel function through endothelial function. Low testosterone is associated with arterial stiffness. There's a tendency toward hypertension with hormone deficiency. Changes occur in blood clotting factors.

How Cardiovascular Disease Affects Hormones

Reduced Blood Flow impairs testicular circulation, thereby affecting hormone production. Many cardiac medications suppress testosterone. Cardiovascular disease limits the benefits of exercise by limiting exercise capacity. Heart disease creates a chronic inflammatory environment.

The Franchise Problem

Franchised men's clinics follow a recipe. Everyone gets treated the same. That's the point of a franchise. Producing identical products through identical practices across all locations. It's the McDonald's model applied to hormone optimization.

But your hormones don't follow a recipe. Your conversion rates are different. Your SHBG levels are different. Your symptoms are different. Your optimal range is different. Cookie-cutter protocols fail because bodies aren't identical.

Many men turn to franchise "men's clinics" that promise quick fixes but often deliver cookie-cutter protocols that overlook individual differences, prioritize sales-focused approaches over medical care, offer limited diagnostic testing, omit crucial factors, employ inexperienced providers without specialized training, and provide no long-term support after initial treatment.

HORMONAL OPTIMIZATION: THE SCIENCE OF RESTORATION

The goal isn't just to achieve "normal" levels; it's to restore optimal function. This requires a sophisticated understanding of hormone interactions and individualized treatment approaches.

Bioidentical Hormone Replacement Therapy (BHRT)

Unlike synthetic hormones, bioidentical hormones have the same molecular structure as those produced by your body.

Advantages of BHRT

Molecular identity refers to the body's recognition and processing of these hormones as natural. Customizable dosing can be tailored to individual needs and response. Multiple delivery methods offer options to suit lifestyles and preferences. Comprehensive monitoring enables regular adjustments based on laboratory results and symptoms. Fewer side effects occur as they're generally better tolerated than synthetic alternatives.

Delivery Method Changes Everything

Most men today receive bioidentical testosterone rather than the older formulations derived from animal sources, such as cows and sheep. That's progress.

But here's what most clinics don't tell you the delivery method fundamentally changes the biochemistry.

Injections convert to estrogen at high rates. Placing the hormone in fat tissue through pellet implants rarely leads to estrogen conversion. Topical testosterone barely penetrates to the blood supply in most men.

I can predict the conversation when a man comes in from another clinic, struggling with side effects from injections.

I ask if their prior provider prescribed an aromatase inhibitor, usually a tiny half tablet taken twice weekly to block estrogen conversion. The answer is always "no."

Then I asked if the first month had been great, but they started crying during the dog food commercials. The answer is always "yes."

That's estrogen conversion. We prevent it, and a month later, they're loving the results.

Delivery Methods: Choosing the Right Approach

Testosterone Injections	
Pros	Precise dosing, cost-effective, excellent absorption, proven track record
Cons	Requires weekly administration, potential for mood swings with peaks/valleys Best for Men who prefer control and don't mind regular injections
Typical Protocol	Weekly subcutaneous or intramuscular injections
Testosterone Pellets	
Pros	Long-lasting (3-4 months), steady hormone levels, convenient
Cons	Minor procedure required, difficult to adjust quickly if needed Best for Men who travel frequently or prefer minimal maintenance
Procedure	Simple office procedure every 3-4 months
Topical Gels/Creams	
Pros	Daily control, easy to adjust dosing, non-invasive
Cons	Transfer risk to partners/children, variable absorption, daily application Best for Men who prefer daily control and want to avoid injections
Application	Applied to the skin daily, usually in the morning and evening

SUPPORTING THERAPIES: THE COMPLETE PICTURE

Estrogen Management

Many men need aromatase inhibitors to prevent excessive testosterone conversion to estrogen. Anastrozole is the most commonly used aromatase inhibitor. Regular estradiol testing helps maintain a proper balance by monitoring. Too little estrogen causes joint pain and mood issues, requiring balance. Individual needs vary... some men need estrogen management, others don't.

Thyroid Optimization

Often overlooked but crucial for energy and metabolism. T4 replacement is standard treatment for hypothyroidism. T3 supplementation may be needed for optimal function. Many patients benefit from combination therapy using both T4 and T3. Regular testing of multiple thyroid markers is essential for monitoring.

Growth Hormone Support

Peptide therapy can stimulate the body's natural production of growth hormone. Sleep optimization is critical since most growth hormone is produced during deep sleep. Resistance training exercise naturally stimulates growth hormone. Adequate protein nutrition and minimal late-night eating support production.

THE PRODUCTIVITY REVELATION

When I started optimizing hormones decades ago, I expected to see improvements in libido, muscle mass, energy, and mood.

What I didn't expect was productivity.

Men report dramatic increases in their ability to accomplish tasks. Focus improves. Mental clarity returns. Projects that felt overwhelming become manageable.

Now I expect to hear about productivity gains at the first follow-up visit. And I do, consistently.

This suggests that testosterone affects cognitive function and motivation beyond physical energy. It's restoring mental capacity that men didn't even realize they'd lost.

THE BILTMORE RESTORATIVE MEDICINE APPROACH TO HORMONE OPTIMIZATION

At Biltmore Restorative Medicine & Aesthetics, our hormone restoration program represents the gold standard of care.

Initial Evaluation Process

Comprehensive Medical History

Detailed evaluation of all symptoms and their impact through symptom assessment, complete review of past health issues and treatments in medical history, evaluation of all current medications and supplements through medication review, diet, exercise, sleep, stress, and environmental factors in lifestyle analysis, and genetic predispositions and family health patterns in family history.

Physical Examination

Thorough head-to-toe assessment in the complete physical, blood pressure, weight, and body composition in vitals and measurements, size, consistency, and any abnormalities in testicular exam, digital rectal exam when appropriate for prostate assessment, and assessment of cardiovascular, neurological, and other systems for overall health.

Advanced Laboratory Testing

Our comprehensive panel far exceeds what most doctors order, including all relevant hormones (not just testosterone) in the complete hormone panel, blood sugar, insulin, lipids, and liver function in metabolic markers, key vitamins and minerals in nutritional assessment, indicators of chronic inflammation in inflammatory markers, and specialized tests based on individual presentation and risk factors.

Treatment Customization

Individual Protocols

Every treatment plan is unique, with no cookie-cutter approaches. It's goal-oriented, based on your specific symptoms and objectives. Lifestyle integration designs treatment to fit your life and schedule. Flexibility allows adjustment as needs change.

Regular Monitoring

Quarterly lab work provides regular testing to ensure optimal levels of performance. Symptom tracking measures both objective and subjective improvement. Regular assessment of treatment effects through physical exams and dosage adjustments involves fine-tuning based on response and lab results.

Lifestyle Integration

Nutrition counseling provides specific recommendations for hormone support. Exercise protocols are designed to enhance hormone production. Stress management encompasses techniques that help reduce cortisol levels and support testosterone production. Sleep optimization provides strategies to improve sleep quality and regulate hormone production.

Ongoing Support

Direct Access

- Direct contact with our medical team for provider communication.
- No concern is too small to discuss when questions are answered.

- A rapid response to any problems or concerns addresses urgent issues and supports ongoing learning about your treatment and health through education.

Educational Resources

- A comprehensive explanation of protocols helps with understanding your treatment.
- Ways to Enhance Treatment Effectiveness through Optimization Strategies.
- Long-term strategies for continued success in health maintenance.
- Updates on new treatments and research for the latest advances.

Real Patient Results:
The Power of Proper Optimization

The transformation possible with proper hormone optimization is remarkable. Here's what one recent patient shared

"I was already losing weight, over 20 pounds, but I was still tired, had little sexual interest or libido, no motivation or focus, and my erections were pitiful! My progress in the gym had plateaued, no matter what I did. I worked out harder and longer, but nothing more was being accomplished!

I had heard great things about the program at Biltmore Restorative Medicine and how much better it was than these franchised 'men's clinics' popping up everywhere, with their commissioned sales tactics and bait-and-switch tactics. I finally decided to contact them. I'm so glad that I did!

They tested for more than just my total testosterone, which my primary care physician had done, and told me my levels were 'fine, that they were within the range.' Doctor Ibrahim showed me that only the lowest 2.5% of labs are labeled 'low' and that, while my level of 322 was within the 'range,' it was literally in the bottom 5th percentile for men! That's low! But no one else could see that but them!

I started on testosterone implants, and within a couple of weeks, my energy was back to its old self, my erections became impressive, and my motivation soared! My muscle mass and strength began to improve again. I lost even more fat and looked 20 years younger, I must say!"

This story illustrates several key points.

- Symptoms matter more than numbers in the "normal" range
- Comprehensive testing reveals what basic tests miss
- Expert interpretation is crucial for proper diagnosis
- Restoration of quality of life extends far beyond sexual function

This patient's journey exemplifies the transformative power of comprehensive hormonal restoration, not just treatment, but true optimization that addresses the root causes and individual needs.

The proper treatment can produce dramatic, life-changing results.

THE SAFETY QUESTION

Here's what I wish the broader medical community would finally understand about testosterone optimization

It's safe to do.

When done correctly, through comprehensive testing, individualized protocols, and ongoing monitoring, hormone optimization is one of the safest interventions in medicine.

The risks come from ignorance, not from the treatment itself. From doctors who don't conduct comprehensive tests. From clinics that use standardized protocols. From providers who don't monitor conversion rates or adjust based on individual response.

At Biltmore Restorative Medicine, we've been optimizing hormones since 2013. We've seen thousands of men transform their lives. Not because we're doing something radical. Because we're doing something thorough.

SAFETY AND MONITORING: THE RESPONSIBLE APPROACH

Proper hormone optimization requires ongoing medical supervision and careful monitoring.

Regular Monitoring Protocol

Laboratory Surveillance

Ensuring optimal ranges for all relevant hormones through hormone level testing, monitoring for any potential side effects through safety markers, PSA testing and physical examination for prostate health, cholesterol, blood pressure, and inflammatory markers for cardiovascular markers, and ensuring healthy red blood cell production through blood counts.

Clinical Assessment

Tracking both objective and subjective changes through symptom improvement, regular assessment of treatment effects with physical examination, monitoring progress toward treatment objectives for goal achievement, and overall life satisfaction and well-being assessment for quality of life.

Potential Risks and Management

Prostate Considerations

Regular PSA testing and examination as part of the screening protocol, evaluation of prostate cancer risk factors in risk assessment, increased vigilance in higher-risk patients through a monitoring strategy, and adjustments if concerns arise through treatment modifications.

Cardiovascular Monitoring

Regular monitoring and management of blood pressure, tracking and optimization of lipid profiles for cholesterol levels, assessment of cardiovascular risk through inflammatory markers, and attention to diet, exercise, and stress management for lifestyle factors.

Blood Count Surveillance

Monitoring for an excessive increase in red blood cell production, ensuring safe levels (target <50%) for hematocrit levels, and donating blood when needed to maintain healthy levels. Additionally, ensure adequate hydration.

THE FUTURE OF HORMONE OPTIMIZATION

The field of hormone optimization continues to evolve with new advances.

Emerging Technologies

Peptide therapy offers more targeted approaches to hormone stimulation. Precision medicine uses genetic testing to guide treatment decisions.

Advanced monitoring uses continuous glucose monitors to track hormone levels. AI-assisted treatment optimization enables personalized protocols.

Research Developments

New delivery methods provide more convenient and effective administration. Combination therapies determine optimal hormone combinations for different patients. Preventive approaches start optimization before symptoms develop. Longevity medicine incorporates hormones into comprehensive anti-aging strategies.

Beyond Normal

The medical system is based on "normal" ranges that encompass 95% of the population.

But normal isn't optimal.

Normal is surviving. Optimal is thriving.

You don't have to accept diminished function just because a lab report says you're within range. Restoration is possible. You don't have to live with symptoms that are destroying your quality of life.

Your body knows the difference between normal and optimal, even if the medical system doesn't.

The question isn't whether your testosterone is "normal" by statistical standards.

The question is whether you feel like yourself.

If the answer is no, and you're struggling with symptoms that are impacting your work, relationships, and sense of vitality, then it's time to look beyond those reference ranges.

It's time to find out what optimal actually feels like.

THE BOTTOM LINE OF YOUR HORMONAL FUTURE

Hormonal decline is inevitable, but you don't have to accept it as part of aging. With proper evaluation, treatment, and monitoring, you can restore hormonal function to optimal levels and regain your vitality.

The key is working with an experienced physician who understands the complexity of hormone optimization and can provide comprehensive, personalized care. At Biltmore Restorative Medicine, we've helped thousands of men feel like themselves again - energetic, confident, and fully engaged in life.

Key Takeaways

- Hormones are complex. Multiple systems work together
- Symptoms matter. More important than being in "normal" range
- Comprehensive testing: Essential for proper diagnosis and treatment
- Individualized treatment: No one-size-fits-all approaches
- Ongoing monitoring: Required for safe and effective treatment
- Expert guidance: Crucial for optimal results

Your hormones are the foundation of your health, energy, and vitality. When optimized correctly, they can help you not just feel better, but feel better than you have in years.

And that requires more than being "normal."

The question isn't whether hormone optimization works... thousands of successful patients prove it does. The question is whether you're ready to take the first step toward restoring your hormonal health and masculine vitality.

At Biltmore Restorative Medicine & Aesthetics, we're here to guide you every step of the way, from comprehensive evaluation to personalized treatment and ongoing optimization. We understand that your hormones aren't just numbers on a lab report. They're the chemical messengers that determine how you feel, how you perform, and how you experience life.

When those messengers are optimized, everything changes, energy returns. Mental clarity sharpens. Muscle builds more easily. Fat melts away. Libido resurges. Confidence rebuilds. Productivity soars.

This isn't about turning back the clock or fighting nature. It's about recognizing that we've already surpassed nature's limitations by living decades beyond our evolutionary design, and now we need to support our bodies in maintaining optimal function throughout that extended lifespan.

Your hormonal future doesn't have to mirror your hormonal present. With the right knowledge, the proper testing, the right treatment, and the right ongoing support, you can feel like yourself again… or perhaps better than you've felt in years.

The choice is yours. Continue accepting "normal" and living with diminished function. Or pursue optimal and restore the vitality that's rightfully yours.

We're here when you're ready to make that choice.

References

Kloner RA.
Erectile dysfunction as a predictor of cardiovascular disease.
Int J Impot Res. 2008;20(5)460-465. PMID 18480824
https//pubmed.ncbi.nlm.nih.gov/18480824/

Dong JY, Zhang YH, Qin LQ.
Erectile dysfunction and risk of cardiovascular disease meta-analysis of prospective cohort studies.
J Am Coll Cardiol. 2011;58(13)1378-1385. PMID 21920268
https//pubmed.ncbi.nlm.nih.gov/21920268/

Jackson G.
Prevention of cardiovascular disease by the early identification of erectile dysfunction
Int J Impot Res. 2008;20 Suppl 2S9-14. PMID 19002117
https//pubmed.ncbi.nlm.nih.gov/19002117/

Gandaglia G, Briganti A, Jackson G, et al.
A systematic review of the association between erectile dysfunction and cardiovascular disease.
Eur Urol. 2014;65(5)968-978. PMID 24011423
https//pubmed.ncbi.nlm.nih.gov/24011423/

CHAPTER 3

Comprehensive Male Enhancement: Beyond the Myths to Real Solutions

WHY MALE ENHANCEMENT FINALLY BECAME MEDICAL SCIENCE

I saw several men lose their penis to untrained providers.

As a practicing urologist, I witnessed catastrophic outcomes from penile enhancement procedures performed by people who had no grasp of anatomy. Men came to me after the damage was done, hoping I could fix what should never have happened in the first place.

I never imagined I'd one day offer penile enhancement myself.

But those failures taught me something critical. This field didn't need to be abandoned. It needed to be done safely, by physicians who understood the anatomy and the science.

That realization changed the trajectory of my practice and ultimately led to the opening of Biltmore Restorative Medicine in 2013.

Understanding Male Enhancement in the Modern Era

After three decades of treating men's sexual health concerns, I've witnessed the evolution of male enhancement from questionable procedures and dubious products to scientifically backed, medically supervised treatments that deliver real results. At Biltmore Restorative Medicine & Aesthetics, we've pioneered approaches that combine the latest advances in regenerative medicine with time-tested urological expertise.

The term "male enhancement" unfortunately carries baggage from years of false advertising and ineffective products. When most men hear it, they think of late-night TV commercials promising unrealistic results from pills or devices that don't work. The reality is far different. Today's evidence-based enhancement treatments are sophisticated medical procedures performed by qualified physicians using FDA-approved products. The products are FDA-approved but used "off-label" for the face; their approval means they are safe and effective. I'm just using them in different areas of the body, which is totally acceptable in the practice of medicine and is not unusual at all.

What Separates Safe Enhancement from Catastrophic Outcomes

Knowing the anatomy is everything.

As a urologist, I operated in that area for years. I understand the vascular structures, the nerve pathways, and the tissue planes. That knowledge prevents the disasters I witnessed early in my career.

The providers who caused those catastrophic outcomes didn't have anatomical expertise. They had marketing materials and aggressive sales tactics.

This is why male enhancement needed to be restored to medical practice. Not because the concept was flawed, but because the execution was dangerous in the hands of untrained users.

When performed by qualified physicians with extensive anatomical knowledge and experience in performing invasive procedures, these treatments are remarkably safe. We're using the patient's own blood. We're applying acoustic energy that's been studied for decades. We're using dermal fillers that have extensive safety profiles.

The difference between safe enhancement and catastrophic outcomes hinges on expertise and ethical practice.

Safe enhancement is about restoring confidence and function through medical science, not marketing gimmicks.

REDEFINING MALE ENHANCEMENT: A COMPREHENSIVE APPROACH

True male enhancement goes far beyond simple size increases. It encompasses a holistic approach to optimizing every aspect of male sexual health and function.

What Actually Matters in Male Enhancement

Most men come in focused on the wrong thing.

They want length. I have to tell them the truth; nothing increases erect penile length. They usually agree because they've already spent money on products that promised results and delivered nothing.

What we can enhance and what we can restore matter.

Erectile quality. Firmness, reliability, endurance. PRP improves this. Acoustic waves improve this. These are the functional improvements that transform sexual experiences.

Girth. Dermal fillers provide visible, measurable enhancement. Partners notice. But here's what I've learned from years of patient feedback: Partners will take firmness over size any day.

Sensitivity. PRP enhances nerve function. Men report heightened sensation without losing control.

Premature ejaculation control. Neurotoxins like Botox decrease retraction and improve endurance. This addresses a problem that affects confidence as much as physical function.

The three dimensions of complete enhancement are functional, physical, and psychological. You can't separate them.

COMPREHENSIVE SEXUAL OPTIMIZATION COMPONENTS

Functional Enhancement

Patients experience enhanced erectile quality with firmer, more sustainable erections. Endurance enhancement provides longer-lasting sexual performance. Sensitivity optimization occurs through improved nerve function and sensation. Response improvement delivers faster arousal and better sexual response, and recovery enhancement results in shorter refractory periods between sexual encounters.

Physical Enhancement

Size optimization includes girth improvements where appropriate. Appearance enhancement provides an improved appearance, both flaccid and erect. Proportional balance ensures natural, proportional results. Texture improvement enhances skin quality and appearance. These physical improvements boost confidence through their psychological benefits.

Performance Confidence

Patients gain psychological benefits, including improved self-image and sexual confidence. Enhanced relationships develop with greater intimacy and partner satisfaction. Reduced anxiety comes through decreased performance anxiety and worry. Improved social confidence extends across all areas of life. Overall well-being improves, as indicated by enhanced quality of life and life satisfaction.

THE SCIENCE BEHIND MODERN ENHANCEMENT

Anatomical Understanding: The Foundation of Effective Treatment

To understand how modern enhancement works, you need to understand penile anatomy.

Penile Structure

The penis consists of three main chambers. The Corpora Cavernosa are two cylindrical chambers that fill with blood during erection. The Corpus Spongiosum surrounds the urethra and forms the glans or head. The Tunica Albuginea is a tough fibrous covering that contains the erectile chambers.

Blood Flow Mechanics

Erection is fundamentally a vascular event. Blood flows into the penis through the penile arteries, creating arterial inflow. Veins are compressed, trapping blood and restricting venous outflow. This process creates rigidity and expansion through pressure increase. The nervous system coordinates the entire process through neurological control.

Enhancement Mechanisms

Modern enhancement techniques improve blood flow and enhance vascular capacity and function. These techniques optimize tissue health by regenerating and strengthening penile tissues. They increase capacity by expanding blood storage. They also enhance nerve function, improving sensitivity and sexual response.

THE ROLE OF GROWTH FACTORS

One of the most significant advances in male enhancement has been the understanding of growth factors and their role in tissue regeneration.

Key Growth Factors

PDGF, or Platelet-Derived Growth Factor, stimulates cell division and blood vessel formation. VEGF, or Vascular Endothelial Growth Factor, promotes the growth of new blood vessels. EGF, or Epidermal Growth Factor, enhances tissue healing and regeneration. FGF, or Fibroblast Growth Factor, supports tissue repair and regeneration. TGF-, or Transforming Growth Factor, regulates cell growth and differentiation.

Natural Healing Process

Your body naturally produces these growth factors in response to injury or stress. Enhancement treatments harness this natural healing response to improve sexual function and appearance.

The Accidental Discovery That Started Everything

The breakthrough in male sexual health came from an unexpected place. Kidney stones.

Back in my urology days, we broke up kidney stones by placing patients in a giant tub of water. Two large spark plugs in the tub would fire, creating pressure waves that shattered the stones. The procedure was called extracorporeal shock wave lithotripsy.

After the procedure, men would routinely tell me something strange.

"Dang, Doc! I never knew a kidney stone could mess with erections! Ever since you broke up that stone, my erections have been fantastic!"

I'd smile and say, "Hey, we are full service here!" thinking the guy was imagining things.

One day, at a conference, a urologist presented a paper. He'd been hearing the same stories and decided to document them. His presentation was titled "Unexpected Improvement in Erectile Quality Following Extracorporeal Shock Wave Lithotripsy A Review of 24 Patients."

That was the beginning of acoustic wave treatment for sexual health.

The lesson? Medical breakthroughs occur when physicians genuinely listen to patients, rather than dismissing what doesn't fit existing models.

This discovery revolutionized how we think about male sexual health, not as something to accept declining, but as something we can actively restore through medical science.

How Controlled Injury Creates Better Function

The science behind acoustic wave therapy is elegantly simple.

The waves create controlled injuries to vessels and nerves. The body recognizes these injuries and sends signals for repair. Platelets rush to the area carrying growth factors.

Here's what makes it work the body repairs the tissue to a better state than before the injury. We call this iatrogenic injury. Intentional damage that triggers superior healing.

Now we use handheld devices instead of bathtubs and spark plugs. The principle remains the same. We're hijacking the body's natural healing response.

When you combine acoustic waves with PRP therapy, you amplify the effect. PRP is a highly concentrated preparation of platelets extracted from the patient's own blood. We're delivering massive amounts of growth factors directly to the tissue we've intentionally injured.

The body thinks it's responding to trauma. Actually, it's an optimization function.

NON-SURGICAL ENHANCEMENT OPTIONS: THE NEW STANDARD OF CARE

The Evolution From Surgery to Regeneration

I chose regenerative approaches over surgical interventions for a reason.

Minimally invasive procedures, such as those using a patient's own blood or acoustic waves, can dramatically enhance function without the risks associated with surgery. No scalpels. No permanent alterations. No extended recovery periods.

Regenerative medicine utilizes the body's natural healing mechanisms to restore function, rather than forcing change through surgical intervention. This approach aligns with my practice of medicine across all aspects of restorative health.

The field has undergone significant evolution since I opened my practice in 2013. Dermal fillers and various Human Cells and Tissue Products are now commonplace. Both are incredibly safe and extraordinarily effective!

We've moved from crude interventions to sophisticated regenerative protocols. From permanent surgical changes to reversible, adjustable treatments. From ignoring the body's healing capacity to amplifying it.

The dangers of permanent enhancements cannot be overstated. Unlike the reversible treatments now available, permanent procedures leave patients with no recourse when trends change, complications arise, or results fail to meet expectations. Permanent implants can migrate, rupture, or cause chronic inflammation. Irreversible surgical alterations made fashionable in one era often become regrettable disfigurements in the next. What's particularly concerning is that permanent enhancements frequently interfere with the body's natural processes and can complicate or prevent future corrective treatments. This is why the shift toward regenerative, adjustable approaches isn't just about better aesthetics; it's fundamentally about patient safety.

This represents medicine at its best, using scientific understanding to enhance natural processes rather than override them.

The P-Shot® (Priapus Shot) Regenerative Medicine Revolution

As one of the few physicians certified to perform the P-Shot®, I've witnessed transformations that still amaze me after performing thousands of these treatments. The P-Shot® represents a paradigm shift from treating symptoms to actually regenerating and healing tissues.

What is the P-Shot®?

The P-Shot® uses Platelet-Rich Plasma (PRP) derived from your own blood to stimulate tissue regeneration and improve function. It's not a foreign substance or drug. It's your body's own healing factors concentrated and delivered where they're needed most.

THE SCIENCE BEHIND PRP THERAPY

Platelet-Rich Plasma Fundamentals

Your blood contains influential healing factors called platelets, which are responsible for clotting and tissue repair. Platelets contain over 30 growth factors and bioactive proteins. These proteins stimulate the formation of new blood vessels through a process known as angiogenesis. They promote tissue regeneration and healing. They improve nerve function and sensitivity. They enhance natural erectile mechanisms. They reduce inflammation and promote healing. They recruit stem cells to the treatment area.

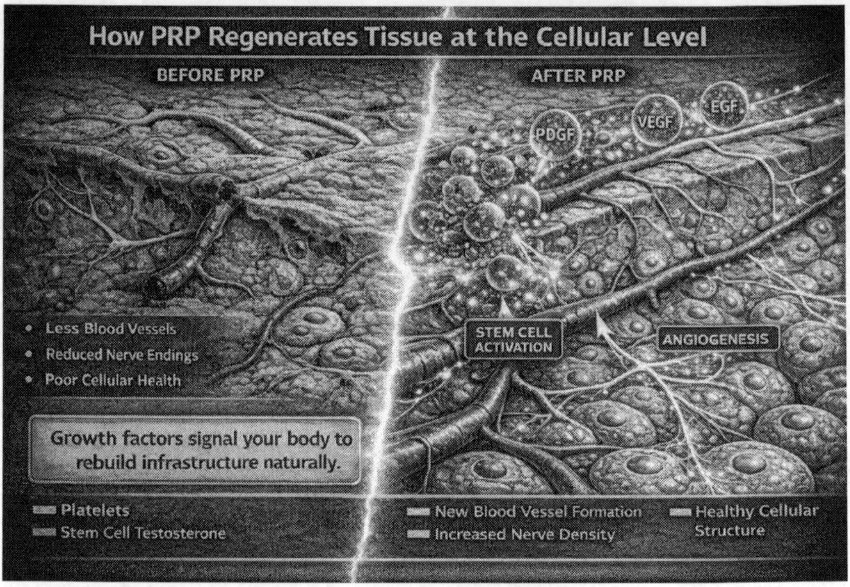

The P-Shot® Procedure Step by Step

Step 1: Blood Collection

We perform a small blood draw of 30-60ml, which is only 1-2 ounces. This is similar to routine lab work. We use specialized collection tubes with an anticoagulant. Sterile technique is maintained throughout the entire process. Patients experience minimal discomfort.

Step 2: PRP Preparation

Blood is processed in a specialized centrifuge. Platelets are concentrated 8-10 times normal levels. This is far greater than most practices, where 1.4 times is the norm, which is less than 2 times! Growth factors are activated for maximum effectiveness.

Step 3: Patient Preparation

Let me be direct, as a urologist, my staff and I know precisely how to numb your penis completely. There is no pain. We use topical numbing cream combined with local anesthetic injections to ensure complete numbness of the treatment area. With proper sterile preparation and comfortable positioning, patients experience no discomfort during the procedure.

Step 4: Strategic Injection

PRP is injected into specific locations with anatomical precision. Several injection points provide optimal coverage through multiple sites. Precise needle placement ensures both safety and effectiveness when using proper technique. We check for any immediate concerns to provide an immediate assessment.

Step 5: Post-Procedure Care

Patients remain for a brief observation period that provides immediate monitoring. We offer detailed post-procedure care guidelines in written instructions. We plan to assess progress by scheduling follow-up appointments. Patients have 24/7 access to our emergency contact for any concerns.

P-SHOT® BENEFITS AND OUTCOMES

Functional Improvements

Enhanced Erectile Quality

Approximately 70-80% of patients report significantly firmer erections. Duration improves with better ability to maintain erections throughout sexual activity. Enhanced natural erectile response without medications provides spontaneity. More reliable erectile function creates consistency. Reduced anxiety about performance builds confidence.

Increased Sensitivity

Growth factors promote nerve healing and function through nerve regeneration. Better sensation during sexual activity enhances pleasure. Heightened awareness improves sexual satisfaction. Enhanced responsiveness increases sexual enjoyment.

Natural Enhancement

Modest but meaningful increases in girth provide size improvement. Enhanced flaccid appearance improves confidence. Improved tissue quality creates better overall aesthetics. Natural-looking results maintain authenticity.

TIMELINE FOR P-SHOT® RESULTS

Initial improvements begin to appear at 2-4 weeks. Significant changes become noticeable between 6 and 8 weeks. Optimal results develop fully by 3 months. Sustained benefits continue for 12-18 months. Maintenance treatments enhance longevity.

Patient Success Story

"Six months after my P-Shot®, I'm performing better than I have in over a decade. My erections are stronger, my sensitivity is incredible, and my confidence is through the roof. My wife and I couldn't be happier with the results. It's like being 25 again, but with the wisdom and experience of my age."

–James, age 48

Why Age Changes the Treatment Approach

Platelets lose growth factors as we age. Our creator wants us to cease to exist eventually. The body's regenerative capacity naturally declines.

This is why I adjust treatment protocols based on age. For patients in their 60s, 70s, or older, I encourage the use of Human Cells and Tissue Products (also known as stem cells) derived from umbilical cord material. These contain far more growth factors than PRP extracted from aged blood.

Exosomes represent the next evolution beyond basic PRP. They're loaded with growth factors that aging platelets can't match.

The science is straightforward: match the treatment to the patient's biological capacity for regeneration. Younger patients respond well to their own concentrated platelets. Older patients benefit from more reliable and comprehensive sources of information.

This isn't one-size-fits-all medicine. It's precision regenerative therapy. This age-adjusted approach ensures optimal outcomes regardless of the patient's biological age, maximizing results while maintaining safety.

P-Shot® Candidacy and Expectations

Ideal Candidates

Patients with mild to moderate erectile dysfunction are most responsive to PRP therapy, showing decreased sensitivity, particularly benefiting from nerve regeneration. Men wanting natural enhancement without surgery are ideal candidates. Those seeking improved sexual performance find excellent results. Men committed to optimizing overall sexual health achieve the best outcomes.

Realistic Expectations

Approximately 70-80% of patients experience significant functional improvement. Nearly universal improvement in sensation and erectile quality occurs. Patient satisfaction rates of over 90% demonstrate effectiveness. Gradual improvement requires patience. Individual results vary based on multiple factors.

Factors Affecting Results

Age plays a role, as younger patients often respond better. Health status matters because overall health affects healing and response. Expectations are essential because realistic expectations are closely tied to satisfaction. Lifestyle factors influence outcomes because habits affect treatment success. Commitment to the protocol is crucial because adherence directly determines the results.

PRIAPUS TOXIN® THE CONFIDENCE GAME-CHANGER

This revolutionary treatment addresses one of men's most common and distressing concerns: penile shrinkage and poor flaccid appearance. Many men are embarrassed by their flaccid size, even when their erect size is perfectly normal.

Understanding Penile Retraction: The Hidden Problem

The Science of Shrinkage

The medical term is "hyperactive penile retraction reflex." This occurs when smooth muscles contract excessively in response to stimuli. Blood flow is restricted to the penis during contraction. The penis retracts closer to the body as a protective mechanism. The flaccid size appears smaller than its actual potential. This response is involuntary and automatic.

Triggers for Penile Retraction

Cold temperatures trigger retraction, including swimming, exposure to cold weather, and use of air conditioning. Stress and anxiety cause retraction through both psychological and physical stress. Physical activity, such as exercise or intense movement during sexual activity, can initiate it. Tight clothing creates pressure and restriction. Fatigue and exhaustion affect muscle tone, triggering retraction.

The "Grower vs. Shower" Dilemma

Many men are "growers" rather than "showers," meaning their flaccid penis appears much smaller than their erectile potential. This can cause locker room anxiety and social discomfort. Partners may initially underestimate size before arousal. Self-consciousness in intimate situations creates psychological distress. First impressions can be misleading and cause concern.

How Priapus Toxin® Works

Mechanism of Action

Similar to the cosmetic applications of neuromodulators, Priapus Toxin works by blocking nerve signals that cause excessive smooth muscle contraction, thereby relaxing smooth muscles in penile tissues. This relaxation improves blood flow to the flaccid penis, maintains a fuller appearance even when not erect, and reduces the shrinkage response to environmental stimuli.

The Science Behind Neuromodulation

Acetylcholine blockade prevents nerve signals that cause muscle contraction. Selective targeting affects only smooth muscles, not erectile function. Controlled relaxation maintains blood flow to the penis. The sustained effect lasts for several months. Reversibility ensures safety because effects are temporary.

Treatment Process: What to Expect

Consultation and Planning

We have a detailed discussion to understand your specific concerns and goals. A physical examination assesses current anatomy and function. Treatment planning customizes the approach to your needs. Setting expectations establishes realistic outcome projections. Pre-procedure instructions prepare you for treatment.

Procedure Day

Local anesthesia produces complete penile numbness. Strategic injection involves precisely placing materials in specific locations. Multiple injection sites ensure comprehensive coverage. The brief procedure duration typically takes 15-20 minutes. Results are typically visible within two weeks after treatment.

Recovery and Timeline

There is no downtime, and patients can return to normal activities immediately. Avoid alcohol 24 hours before and after for optimal results. Initial effects appear within 2-4 weeks. Maximum benefit is typically achieved within 6 to 8 weeks. Results usually last 3-4 months.

EXPECTED OUTCOMES FROM PRIAPUS TOXIN®

Appearance Improvements

Enhanced Girth

The improved circumference throughout provides a fuller appearance. The overall appearance is more substantial and prominent. Enhanced proportions create better aesthetics. Visual impact improves confidence. Natural-looking enhancement maintains authenticity.

Functional Benefits Beyond Appearance

Improved Erectile Function

Enhanced circulation during arousal provides better blood flow. The improved rigidity and sustainability create firmer erections. Decreased retraction maintains a fuller appearance during sex. Better erectile quality enhances sexual performance. Increased confidence reduces performance anxiety.

Enhanced Sexual Performance

For men struggling with premature ejaculation, this represents the only genuine medical intervention available, a breakthrough for a condition that has historically had few effective treatment options. By reducing the hyperactive retraction reflex, Priapus Toxin® can delay ejaculation and improve control. Many patients report significant improvements in their ability to delay ejaculation. This leads to greater sexual satisfaction for both partners. The psychological relief from addressing this concern often further improves overall sexual confidence.

Duration and Maintenance

Noticeable improvement occurs within 2-4 weeks for initial results. The typical duration is 3 to 4 months. Maintenance treatments sustain results over time. Individual variation affects the longevity of results.

Patient Testimonial

"I was always self-conscious in locker rooms and with partners. Priapus Toxin® changed everything. I finally look like the 'shower' I always wanted to be instead of just a 'grower.' The confidence boost has been incredible - it's affected every area of my life, not just sexual situations."

–Mark, age 42

ACOUSTIC WAVE THERAPY REVOLUTION

This FDA-approved technology represents a breakthrough in treating erectile dysfunction and enhancing sexual performance naturally, without drugs or surgery.

The Science of Acoustic Wave Therapy

Low-Intensity Shockwave Technology

Acoustic wave therapy uses focused acoustic waves that break down microplaques in blood vessels. The treatment stimulates the growth of new blood vessels through a process known as neovascularization. It improves the function of existing blood vessels, enhancing circulation. The therapy enhances tissue health and regeneration. Natural healing processes are activated without the use of medications.

Mechanism of Action

- Mechanical stimulation occurs when sound waves induce controlled microtrauma.

- Vasodilation happens when blood vessels dilate, improving circulation.
- Neovascularization occurs when new blood vessels form, thereby increasing blood vessel capacity.
- Tissue remodeling produces improved tissue structure and function.
- Growth factor release activates natural healing factors.

Why Acoustic Wave Therapy Works When Pills Don't

It addresses the root cause by improving actual blood flow rather than just symptoms. These products have no side effects, unlike those commonly found in medications. Long-lasting results persist for months or years. The treatment is drug-free, relying on natural mechanisms. Results are cumulative and improve over time.

Acoustic Wave Therapy Treatment Protocol

Initial Treatment Series

The treatment series consists of 6-12 treatments over 3-6 weeks for optimal frequency. Each session lasts 15-20 minutes. Typically, treatments are scheduled one to two times per week. There is no downtime between sessions. The progressive protocol builds cumulative effects.

Treatment Experience

The patient lies comfortably during the procedure. Acoustic waves are applied to specific areas of the penis. Mild tingling or pulsing sensations may occur. The treatment is well-tolerated with minimal discomfort. Patients can resume normal activities immediately after treatment.

Progressive Results Timeline

Initial improvements in erectile function are seen at 2-4 weeks. Significant changes in firmness and duration develop by 6-8 weeks. Optimal results manifest at 3 months. Sustained benefits continue for 1-2 years. Maintenance treatments extend the longevity of results.

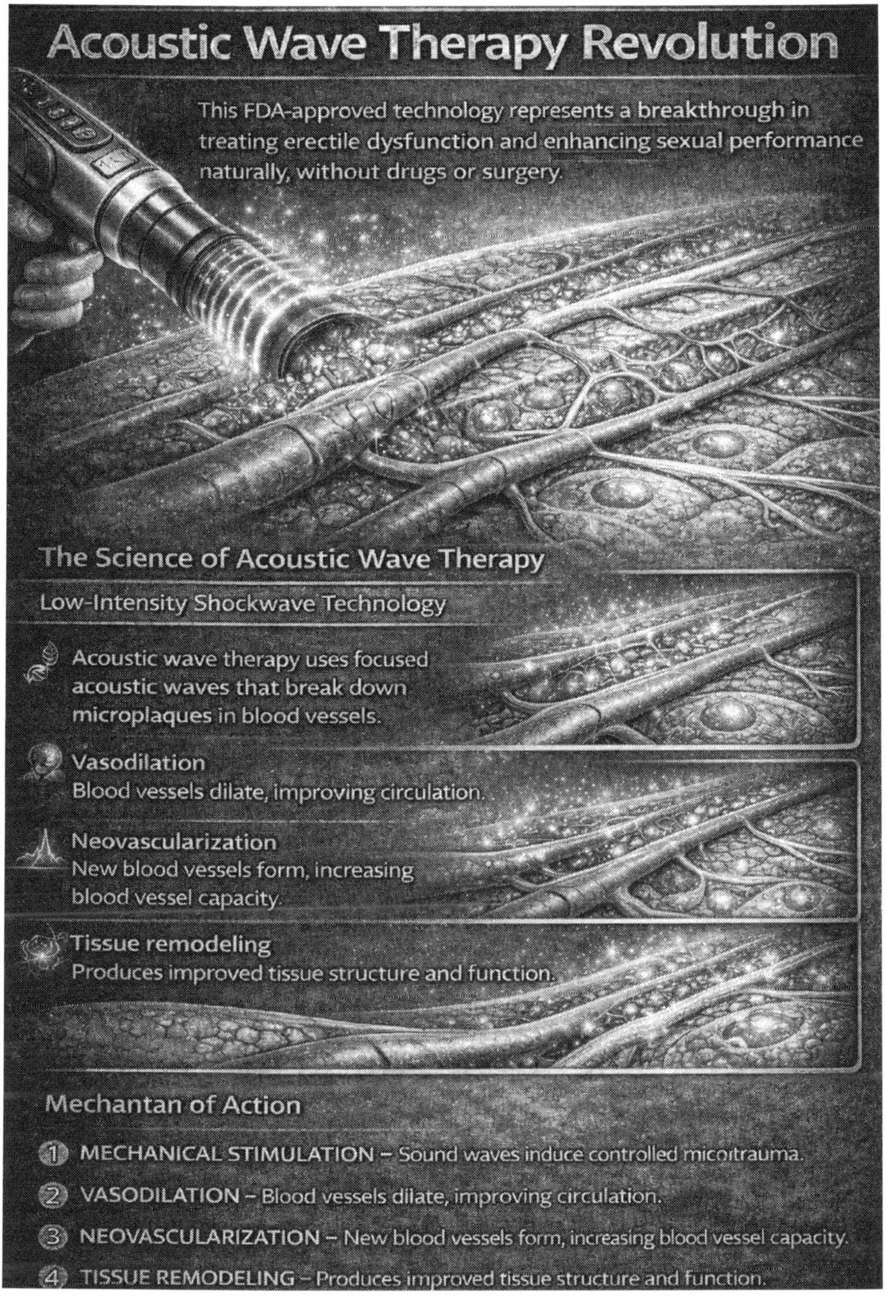
Acoustic Wave Therapy Revolution
This FDA-approved technology represents a breakthrough in treating erectile dysfunction and enhancing sexual performance naturally, without drugs or surgery.
The Science of Acoustic Wave Therapy
Low-Intensity Shockwave Technology
Acoustic wave therapy uses focused acoustic waves that break down microplaques in blood vessels.
Vasodilation
Blood vessels dilate, improving circulation.
Neovascularization
New blood vessels form, increasing blood vessel capacity.
Tissue remodeling
Produces improved tissue structure and function.
Mechantan of Action
1 MECHANICAL STIMULATION – Sound waves induce controlled micoitrauma.
2 VASODILATION – Blood vessels dilate, improving circulation.
3 NEOVASCULARIZATION – New blood vessels form, increasing blood vessel capacity.
4 TISSUE REMODELING – Produces improved tissue structure and function.

ACOUSTIC WAVE THERAPY BENEFITS BEYOND ED TREATMENT

Erectile Function Enhancement

Improved Firmness

Patients experience harder, more sustainable erections with improved rigidity. The erectile response becomes more consistent and reliable. Greater fullness and engorgement occur during arousal. Erections develop faster with quicker response time. Confidence increases from predictable performance.

Enhanced Duration

Erections last longer for better sustainability. Sexual endurance improves for greater stamina. The refractory period decreases with a shorter recovery time. The ability for multiple sexual encounters increases. Overall, sexual vitality enhances satisfaction.

Performance Enhancement Benefits

Increased Sensitivity

Enhanced nerve response and sensation improve nerve function. Sensation and enjoyment become better during sexual activity. Heightened awareness increases pleasure. Improved sensitivity enhances intimate experiences. Better nerve health supports sexual function.

Natural Response

Patients experience reduced dependence on ED medications for drug-free function. The ability for spontaneous sexual activity without planning improves. A more natural sexual response develops over time. Improved confidence grows from knowing the function is reliable. Freedom from medication side effects provides relief.

Patient Success Story

"After my Acoustic Wave Therapy series, I threw away my ED medications. My natural function returned better than it had been in years. The convenience of not needing pills and the spontaneity it brought back to our relationship has been amazing. My wife says it's like having the old me back."

–Robert, age 55

ACOUSTIC WAVE THERAPY VS. OTHER ED TREATMENTS

Advantages Over Medications

This natural process has no drug reactions and produces no side effects. The benefits continue for 1-2 years without daily medication. Treatment addresses underlying causes rather than masking symptoms. Results are sustained without ongoing medication costs. Natural improvement becomes permanent in many cases.

Advantages Over Surgery

There are no surgical risks or complications. The treatment uses the body's own healing mechanisms for natural regeneration. Recovery time is minimal with no downtime required. Results appear natural without artificial implants. The reversible nature provides peace of mind.

RestoreMore Advanced Girth Enhancement

Our proprietary approach to penile girth enhancement represents the evolution of dermal filler techniques applied to male enhancement. Unlike generic "penile filler" procedures, RestoreMore is a sophisticated, physician-designed protocol.

THE RESTOREMORE DIFFERENCE

Why We Developed RestoreMore

Traditional "penile filler" procedures often resulted in unnatural appearance with irregular or disproportionate results. Poor integration occurred, leading to filler migration or the formation of lumps. Limited longevity meant frequent repeat procedures were needed. Safety concerns arose from the use of unqualified providers and non-approved materials. Patient dissatisfaction was common with unpredictable outcomes.

Our Advanced Approach

A board-certified urologist created the physician-designed protocol. We use only FDA-approved materials for maximum safety and reliability. Advanced techniques ensure natural-looking results. Precise injection protocols optimize distribution. Comprehensive patient education sets realistic expectations.

Scientific Foundation

We utilize biocompatible materials to ensure tissue compatibility. Our understanding of how fillers integrate with penile tissue guides our approach. Gradual, controlled enhancement prevents over-correction. Multiple sessions allow for adjustment and refinement. Safety protocols minimize complication risks.

RESTOREMORE PROCEDURE DETAILS

Pre-Procedure Preparation

Comprehensive Consultation

We focus on understanding your specific enhancement objectives through goal assessment. A clear discussion of realistic outcomes establishes appropriate expectations, and before-and-after photos illustrate potential results. A detailed explanation of the procedure prepares you. Opportunity for questions ensures informed decision-making.

Medical Clearance

We conduct a comprehensive medical evaluation to assess overall health. We ensure optimal health status through screening. We review medications and supplements for safety. We assess healing capacity to predict outcomes. We obtain informed consent after a thorough discussion.

The RestoreMore Process

Step 1: Preparation and Anesthesia

We provide local anesthesia for complete comfort through comprehensive numbing. We create a hospital-grade sterile field to prevent infection. We position you correctly for optimal access. We maintain your privacy and dignity throughout. We ensure you are completely comfortable before proceeding.

Step 2: Strategic Enhancement

We identify optimal injection zones through anatomical mapping. We use multiple injection points for even distribution. We employ precise techniques for smooth, natural results. We build gradually to avoid over-correction. We assess immediately for symmetry and appearance.

Step 3: Immediate Post-Procedure Care

We perform an immediate evaluation of the enhancement to assess results. Pain management and swelling control protocols are initiated. You will receive detailed aftercare instructions. We schedule follow-up appointments for monitoring. We provide emergency contact information for concerns.

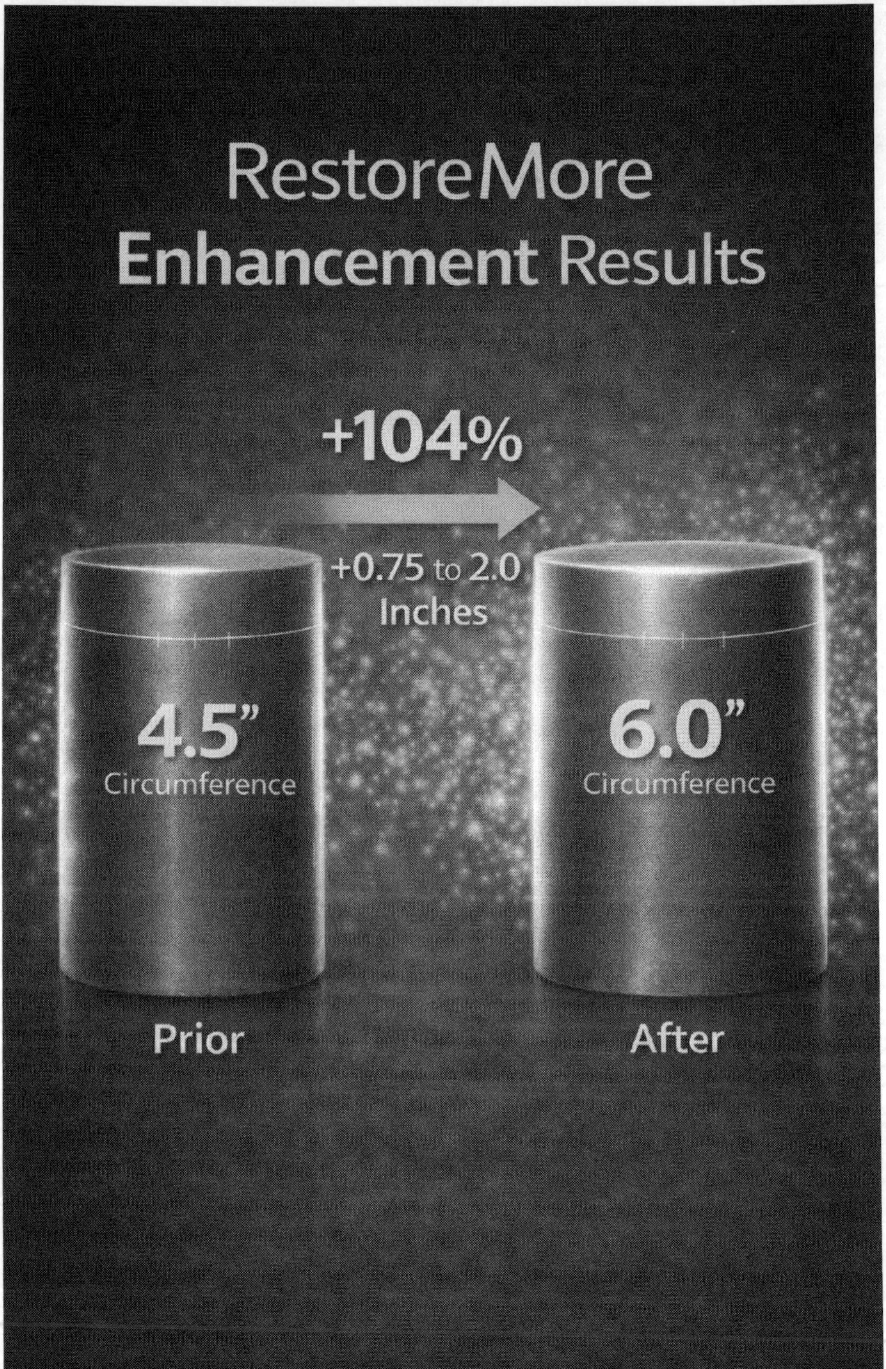
RestoreMore
Enhancement Results
+104%
+0.75 to 2.0
Inches
4.5”
Circumference
6.0”
Circumference
Prior
After

RESTOREMORE RESULTS AND EXPECTATIONS

Enhancement Outcomes

Girth Increase

The mathematics of girth enhancement reveals something remarkable. The average erect penis measures just under 5 inches in length and 4.5 inches in circumference. Increasing circumference by 1.5 inches represents roughly a 104% increase in volume, a dramatic difference. Most patients achieve a 0.75 to 2.0-inch increase in circumference. This translates to an over 100% increase in volume. Visual impact exceeds what the measurements suggest. Partners consistently report noticeable differences.

Quality Results

The soft, natural texture is maintained for a natural feel. Normal sexual function is preserved without interference. Partner satisfaction increases with enhanced girth. Confidence improvements are significant and immediate. Results look and feel entirely natural.

Timeline and Recovery

Immediate Results

Results are visible immediately following the procedure. Patients should expect moderate swelling and minor bruising initially. The initial appearance is slightly larger than the final result. Enhancement settles over the first few weeks. True results become apparent at 2-4 weeks.

Recovery Process

After one week, you can resume normal activities.

Longevity and Maintenance

Typical longevity is 9-12 months, after which additional units are needed to 'top off the tank.' Some patients experience a longer duration due to individual factors. Touch-up treatments maintain optimal results. A gradual enhancement strategy allows for adjustments. Long-term patients achieve stable, sustained enhancement.

THE MAINTENANCE REALITY NOBODY WANTS TO HEAR

The biggest misconception men have about these treatments is that they're permanent. They're not.

Doing one P-shot and never repeating it is like painting a house once. The paint will fade. The protection will diminish. You'll need to repaint.

The same principle applies to regenerative treatments. The benefits won't last indefinitely without maintenance.

This is precisely how I approach hormone optimization in my practice. It's an ongoing commitment to maintaining optimal function, not a quick fix that lasts forever.

Men need to understand this upfront. These treatments work. The results are real and measurable. But maintaining those results requires a schedule of repeat treatments.

I'd rather set realistic expectations than promise permanence I can't deliver.

Understanding this upfront allows patients to make informed decisions and plan for long-term maintenance of their results. It's not a drawback. It's a realistic approach to sustained excellence.

COMBINATION THERAPY: THE SYNERGISTIC APPROACH

The most dramatic and lasting results often occur when multiple treatments are combined in a coordinated, comprehensive protocol.

The Complete Enhancement Protocol

Phase 1: Foundation Building (Weeks 1-4)

We begin with hormone optimization, initiating testosterone replacement if needed. Lifestyle modification is achieved through a combination of diet, exercise, and stress management. We address any underlying health issues that may affect outcomes. We optimize cardiovascular health for better blood flow. We establish baseline measurements for tracking progress.

Phase 2: Regeneration (Weeks 5-12)

The P-Shot® treatment stimulates tissue regeneration and blood flow. Progress monitoring includes regular assessments and adjustments. Acoustic wave therapy is added if appropriate to amplify effects. We track improvements in function and satisfaction. We adjust protocols based on individual response.

Phase 3: Enhancement (Weeks 13-16)

Priapus Toxin® is then administered to optimize both flaccid appearance and overall function. For patients seeking girth enhancement, RestoreMore may be added at this stage. We combine treatments for synergistic effects. We assess cumulative improvements across all parameters. We refine our approach based on the patient's goals and response.

Phase 4: Maintenance (Ongoing)

Regular monitoring includes quarterly check-ups and assessments. Touch-up treatments maintain and enhance initial results. Lifestyle optimization continues to support treatment outcomes. Hormone levels are monitored and adjusted as needed. Long-term relationship supports sustained success.

Synergistic Benefits of Combination Therapy

Enhanced Outcomes

All aspects of sexual health are addressed for comprehensive improvement. Treatments work together for synergistic effects. Results exceed what single treatments achieve on their own. Comprehensive optimization addresses multiple concerns simultaneously. Holistic improvement transforms the overall sexual experience.

Patient Satisfaction Benefits

The combined approach is more effective than individual treatments, resulting in higher success rates. Cost-effectiveness improves through bundled treatment packages. Convenience increases with coordinated scheduling. Long-term value comes from sustained, comprehensive improvements. Patient commitment increases with visible progress.

Real-World Results

Patients who choose comprehensive protocols typically report life-changing improvements. They experience dramatic transformations in both function and confidence. Their relationships improve as intimacy and satisfaction increase. Their overall quality of life increases significantly. They become advocates for a comprehensive approach.

The Confidence That Extends Beyond the Bedroom

Men who become more confident in the bedroom carry that confidence everywhere. At work. At play. In every interaction.

This isn't abstract psychology. I see it in how patients walk into follow-up appointments. How do they make eye contact? How do they talk about their relationships?

Sexual confidence creates a ripple effect through a man's entire life. When you address the root cause of sexual dysfunction instead of masking symptoms, you're not just improving erections. You're restoring a fundamental aspect of how men experience themselves.

Every patient who undergoes these treatments reports satisfaction. Their partners report satisfaction. That's not marketing. That's consistent clinical outcomes.

COMPARING ENHANCEMENT OPTIONS: MAKING THE RIGHT CHOICE NON-SURGICAL VS. SURGICAL APPROACHES

Non-Surgical Advantages

Safety Profile

There is a minimal risk compared to surgery, with lower complication rates. Recovery takes days instead of weeks for a faster return to everyday life. No general anesthesia is needed for safer procedures. Outpatient treatments are convenient for busy schedules. Reversibility provides peace of mind.

Results Quality

These procedures produce more natural-looking outcomes compared to traditional surgical interventions. Adjustable results allow for refinement over time. No permanent alterations preserve natural anatomy. Gradual improvement appears more natural to others. Partner satisfaction is high with realistic enhancement.

Convenience Factors

No hospital stays are required for office procedures. Patients can return to work immediately after same-day treatment. Lower costs compared to surgery make treatment more accessible. Flexible scheduling accommodates busy lifestyles. A less invasive approach reduces anxiety.

When Surgical Options Might Be Considered

Specific Medical Conditions

Severe Peyronie's disease, characterized by severe curvature, may require surgery. Congenital abnormalities requiring reconstruction for birth defects need surgical intervention. Trauma reconstruction after injury or damage may necessitate surgery. A penile prosthesis may be necessary for severe ED when other treatments fail. Specific anatomical issues that cannot be addressed non-surgically could require surgery.

Patient Factors

Failed non-surgical approaches after unsuccessful conservative treatment might warrant surgery. Specific requirements for particular anatomical needs may require surgical solutions. Realistic expectations involve understanding the limitations and risks associated with surgery. A strong preference, despite proper counseling on alternatives, may be appropriate. Medical clearance ensures that the patient can undergo surgery safely.

PATIENT SELECTION AND CANDIDACY

Ideal Candidates for Non-Surgical Enhancement

Candidates should be in good general health and able to heal normally. An absence of active infections or skin conditions in the treatment area is essential. Realistic anatomy means having adequate tissue for treatment. Stable weight prevents fluctuations that affect results. No bleeding disorders ensure safe procedures.

Candidates should have stable mental health without severe psychological disorders. Realistic expectations about outcomes prevent disappointment. Understanding that enhancement is not the same as transformation is crucial. Personal motivation rather than external pressure ensures satisfaction. Emotional stability supports the treatment process.

Candidates must refrain from smoking at least one week prior and after treatment, as tobacco use significantly impairs healing and compromises results. Alcohol consumption should be moderate because excess affects healing. Commitment to healthy lifestyle choices supports optimal outcomes. Following post-procedure instructions ensures proper recovery. Realistic time commitments for follow-up appointments are necessary.

MANAGING EXPECTATIONS: THE KEY TO SATISFACTION

Realistic Outcome Expectations

Enhancement Magnitude

A 20-40% increase in girth is achievable, and an over 100% increase in volume displacement is possible. Most patients experience a significant enhancement, but not a dramatic transformation. Functional improvements are often more impactful than size changes. Individual results vary based on anatomy and technique. Realistic goals lead to higher satisfaction.

Satisfaction Factors

Realistic expectations directly correlate with satisfaction. Provider expertise and experience have a significant impact on outcomes. Patient commitment to the process influences results. Communication between the patient and the provider ensures alignment. Follow-up care maintains and optimizes results.

Factors That Optimize Results

Pre-Treatment Optimization

We optimize overall health before treatment. We address diet, exercise, sleep, and stress management to improve lifestyle. We correct hormonal imbalances to optimize hormone levels. We manage chronic conditions for medical stability. We ensure proper hydration and nutrition to support healing.

Post-Treatment Maintenance

To maintain long-term results, patients should commit to the healthy habits they've developed during treatment. This includes keeping scheduled follow-up appointments for monitoring. As recommended, touch-up therapies sustain optimal results. Ongoing hormone optimization, if applicable, maintains benefits. Continued healthy lifestyle choices support sustained enhancement.

ADVANCED TECHNOLOGIES AND FUTURE INNOVATIONS

The field of male enhancement continues to evolve with exciting new developments on the horizon.

What the Future Holds

I don't have a crystal ball for predicting the next breakthrough.

I believe regenerative medicine will continue to advance. We'll discover more potent sources of growth factors. We'll refine delivery methods. We will gain a better understanding of the cellular mechanisms that drive tissue optimization.

The trajectory is clear away from synthetic interventions and toward treatments that harness the body's innate regenerative capacity.

What I hope changes most is the conversation around male sexual health. This field deserves to be discussed with the same medical legitimacy as any other aspect of health optimization.

Men deserve access to evidence-based treatments performed by qualified physicians. They deserve realistic expectations. They deserve safety.

Emerging Treatment Options

Stem Cell Therapy

Stem cell therapy utilizes the patient's own stem cells for enhancement through autologous cell therapy. It offers greater regenerative potential than standard PRP. Longer-lasting results may be achieved with stem cells. Enhanced tissue regeneration is achieved through stem cell therapy. Research continues to expand applications.

Growth Factor Concentrates

Growth factor concentrates are more potent than standard platelet preparations, as they are enhanced PRP. They offer a higher concentration of active healing factors. Improved outcomes may result in some patients. Advanced processing techniques yield better preparations. Emerging as a next-generation enhancement option.

Peptide Therapy

Peptide therapy uses specific peptides for sexual health as targeted healing. It includes peptides that enhance tissue repair and regeneration. Combinations with other treatments amplify effects. Oral or injectable administration provides flexibility. Research continues to identify effective peptides.

Technology Advancement Areas

Improved Delivery Systems

Modern injection systems have revolutionized the administration of treatments. These advanced delivery systems improve precision and reduce discomfort. Microneedling devices enhance product penetration and absorption. Automated injection systems ensure consistent dosing and distribution. Novel delivery methods continue to emerge, improving outcomes.

Enhanced Monitoring

Today's monitoring technology enables healthcare providers to evaluate treatment effects in real-time. Ultrasound technology objectively assesses blood flow and tissue changes. Standardized measurements track progress with consistency. Patient-reported outcomes capture subjective improvements. Comprehensive data guides treatment adjustments and optimization.

The Bottom Line: Your Enhancement Journey

At Biltmore Restorative Medicine & Aesthetics, we're committed to restoring your sexual health and confidence safely and effectively. Our combination of urological expertise, advanced technology, and personalized care ensures the best possible outcomes for our patients.

That's what three decades in medicine taught me. And that's what drives my practice at Biltmore Restorative Medicine.

Male enhancement isn't about late-night commercials and questionable products anymore. It's about medical science, regenerative healing, and comprehensive sexual health optimization.

That transformation didn't happen by accident. It happened because physicians started listening to patients, understanding the science, and offering treatments that actually work.

Remember, true enhancement isn't just about size; it's about optimizing every aspect of your sexual health and confidence to help you feel like the best version of yourself. The comprehensive approach we offer addresses not just physical enhancement, but function, confidence, and overall sexual wellness.

Key Principles of Our Approach

Medical Excellence

We offer advanced urological expertise, backed by decades of experience. We exclusively use FDA-approved technologies and materials. Continuous education keeps us current with the latest advances. An evidence-based approach ensures proven treatments.

Individualized Care

Every patient receives a customized treatment plan tailored to their specific needs and goals, with no cookie-cutter approaches. Thorough assessment identifies optimal treatment strategies. Flexible protocols adapt to individual response and progress. Direct physician involvement throughout ensures the delivery of quality care. Personalized attention addresses unique concerns.

Regenerative Focus

Our approach harnesses your body's natural healing capacity whenever possible, using your own biological materials. Minimally invasive techniques minimize risk and downtime. Natural-looking results maintain an authentic appearance. Reversible treatments provide flexibility and peace of mind. Enhancement without permanent alteration preserves options.

Comprehensive Support

You'll have direct access to our experienced medical team throughout your treatment journey. Through regular monitoring, protocol adjustments, and thorough follow-up care, we ensure optimal outcomes. Clear communication keeps you informed at every step. Supportive environment addresses concerns compassionately. Long-term partnership supports sustained success.

WHAT SETS BILTMORE RESTORATIVE MEDICINE APART

Expertise and Safety

As a urologist with over 30 years of experience, I bring anatomical knowledge that prevents the catastrophic outcomes I witnessed early in my career. Hospital-grade sterile protocols ensure infection prevention. Conservative approach prioritizes safety over aggressive enhancement. Proper training in advanced procedures guarantees competence. Track record of safety speaks for itself.

Honest Communication

I tell patients the truth about what works and what doesn't. Length enhancement isn't realistic, so I don't promise it. What we can deliver, improved firmness, sensitivity, control, and modest girth increases, I stand behind completely. Being transparent about limitations builds trust. Honesty about realistic outcomes prevents disappointment.

Evidence-Based Practice

We don't chase trends or offer unproven treatments. Every procedure we perform has scientific backing, clinical data, and a track record of safety and efficacy. Published research supports our methods. Peer-reviewed studies validate our approaches. Continuous evaluation ensures quality standards.

Realistic Expectations

I'd rather have a patient walk away disappointed that we can't promise miracles than have them undergo treatment with false expectations. This honest approach attracts patients who value truth over marketing. Satisfaction rates are higher when expectations align with reality. Trust is built on transparency, not exaggeration.

THE COMPLETE PICTURE

Enhancement is one piece of the larger restoration picture. It works best when combined with

Hormonal Optimization

Testosterone and other hormones at optimal levels provide the foundation for sexual function. No amount of enhancement will compensate for hormonal deficiencies. Comprehensive hormone testing identifies imbalances affecting sexual health. Replacement therapy restores hormonal balance when needed. Ongoing monitoring maintains optimal levels.

Lifestyle Optimization

Good nutrition, regular exercise, quality sleep, and stress management all enhance treatment outcomes and sustain results in the long term. Cardiovascular health directly affects erectile function and treatment response. Weight management improves outcomes and overall health. Stress reduction enhances sexual performance and satisfaction. Holistic health supports comprehensive wellness.

Relationship Health

Sexual function is often experienced within the context of relationships. Addressing communication, intimacy, and emotional connection enhances outcomes beyond physical treatments alone. Partner involvement in the treatment process can improve success. Relationship counseling may complement physical therapies. A holistic approach considers all aspects of sexual health.

MAKING YOUR DECISION

Choosing to pursue enhancement treatments is a significant decision. Here's what you should consider

Evaluate Your Motivation

Are you seeking enhancement for yourself or to please someone else? The most satisfied patients pursue treatment for their own confidence and satisfaction, not to meet someone else's expectations. Internal motivation predicts better outcomes and satisfaction. Personal goals should drive treatment decisions. Self-improvement focus leads to lasting benefits.

Assess Your Expectations

Can you be satisfied with modest but meaningful improvements? Or are you seeking dramatic transformations that aren't realistic? Understanding what's achievable prevents disappointment. Realistic goals lead to higher satisfaction. Dramatic changes typically aren't possible or advisable.

Consider the Commitment

Are you prepared for the maintenance that sustained results require? These aren't one-time procedures but ongoing commitments to optimal sexual health. Long-term success requires sustained effort and investment. Maintenance treatments preserve and enhance initial results. Lifestyle optimization supports lasting benefits.

Choose Your Provider Carefully

Credentials matter, experience matters. Honesty matters. The provider you choose will significantly impact your outcomes and safety. Research providers thoroughly before making decisions. Verify credentials and experience in the specific procedures. Seek providers who prioritize safety over profit. Trust your instincts when evaluating a provider's competence and integrity.

YOUR NEXT STEPS

If you're considering enhancement, the first step is a comprehensive consultation. During this visit, we'll:

Understand Your Goals

What specific concerns are you trying to address? What outcomes would represent success for you? What aspects of your sexual health most affect your confidence and satisfaction? Clarifying goals guides treatment planning. Defining success ensures alignment of expectations. Understanding priorities optimizes treatment strategy.

Assess Your Current Status

We conduct a comprehensive physical examination to gain a thorough understanding of your anatomy. We review your medical history and current health status. We perform lab work if needed to assess overall health. We evaluate baseline sexual function for comparison. We identify factors that may affect treatment outcomes.

Develop Your Plan

We create a customized treatment protocol based on your specific needs. We provide a clear explanation of expected outcomes and timeline. We discuss potential risks and outline the measures we take to mitigate them. We outline costs and payment options transparently. We establish a follow-up schedule for monitoring progress.

Set Expectations

We have an honest conversation about what's achievable and what's not. Discussion of potential risks and how we minimize them occurs openly. The timeline for results is clearly and realistically explained. Maintenance requirements for sustained benefits are outlined. Alternativc options are presented if appropriate.

The Transformation Is Real

I've performed thousands of these procedures over the past decade. The transformations I've witnessed aren't just physical; they're psychological, relational, and existential.

Men walk differently after successful enhancement. They make eye contact. They engage in activities they'd been avoiding. They report improved work performance, better relationships, and enhanced overall life satisfaction.

This isn't hyperbole. This is what happens when you address a source of shame, anxiety, or inadequacy with adequate medical treatment.

The confidence that comes from improved sexual function radiates into every area of life. It's not vanity. It's reclaiming a fundamental aspect of masculine identity and wellbeing.

A FINAL WORD ON SAFETY

Everything we do at Biltmore Restorative Medicine is grounded in safety first.

We use only FDA-approved materials and technologies. We maintain hospital-grade sterile protocols. We conduct comprehensive patient screening prior to treatment. We provide detailed informed consent. We keep meticulous procedural documentation.

Most importantly, we know when to say no. Not every patient is a good candidate. Not every desired outcome is achievable. Not every request is in the patient's best interest. Ethical practice sometimes means declining to treat a patient. Patient safety always takes precedence over profit.

This commitment to safety distinguishes us from providers who view enhancement as a profit center rather than a medical practice. Your safety and satisfaction are always our top priority.

THE INVITATION

Your journey to enhanced sexual health and confidence begins with a conversation.

We understand that reaching out takes courage. Many men suffer in silence for years before seeking help. The shame and embarrassment that surround sexual concerns keep men from accessing treatments that could transform their lives.

But you don't have to continue suffering. You don't have to accept decline as inevitable. You don't have to settle for less than optimal sexual function. Solutions exist that can help restore your confidence and vitality. Professional help is available when you're ready.

Effective treatments exist. Qualified physicians can help. Real transformations are possible. The science is sound and proven. The results speak for themselves.

The question isn't whether these treatments work; thousands of satisfied patients prove they do. The question is whether you're ready to take the first step toward restoring your sexual vitality and confidence. We're here to help when you decide the time is right.

The question is whether you're ready to take the first step toward restoring your sexual vitality and confidence.

We're here when you are.

At Biltmore Restorative Medicine & Aesthetics, we've helped thousands of men achieve the sexual function, appearance, and confidence they deserve. We combine decades of urological expertise with the latest advances in regenerative medicine to deliver safe, effective, and life-changing results.

This field has evolved from questionable procedures to legitimate medical science. From empty promises to documented outcomes. From dangerous experimentation to evidence-based protocols.

That evolution occurred because physicians like me chose to restore this field to legitimate medical practice, practicing it with the expertise, ethics, and evidence that all medicine should embody.

You deserve that level of care. You deserve honest communication, realistic expectations, and treatments that actually work. You deserve a provider who prioritizes your safety and satisfaction above all else. You deserve expertise backed by decades of experience.

Your enhancement journey starts here. We look forward to helping you achieve your goals and experience the confidence that comes with optimal sexual function. Contact us today to schedule your confidential consultation. Take the first step toward the transformation you deserve.

Because at the end of the day, this isn't just about enhancement. It's about restoring a fundamental aspect of your masculine identity and living life with the confidence, vitality, and satisfaction you deserve.

References

Dr. Paul Perito
Perito Urology
Developer of UroFill®
https://peritourology.com/

Poulios E, Mykoniatis I, Pyrgidis N, et al.
Platelet-Rich Plasma (PRP) Improves Erectile Function A Double-Blind, Randomized, Placebo-Controlled Clinical Trial.
J Sex Med. 2021;18(5)926-935. PMID 33906807
https//pubmed.ncbi.nlm.nih.gov/33906807/

Shaher H, Fathi A, Elbashir S, et al.
Is Platelet Rich Plasma Safe and Effective in Treatment of Erectile Dysfunction? Randomized Controlled Study.
Urology. 2023;175114-119.
PMID 36736914
https//pubmed.ncbi.nlm.nih.gov/36736914/

Zhang J, Xiong J, Fang J, et al.
The efficacy of platelet rich plasma in the treatment of erectile dysfunction a systematic review and meta-analysis.
Andrologia. 2024;56(5)e15745.
PMID 38832665
https//pubmed.ncbi.nlm.nih.gov/38832665/

Poulios E, Mykoniatis I, Pyrgidis N, et al.
Platelet-rich plasma for the treatment of erectile dysfunction a systematic review of preclinical and clinical studies.
Sex Med Rev. 2023;11(4)359-368.
PMID 37528499
https//pubmed.ncbi.nlm.nih.gov/37528499/

CHAPTER 4

Are You Ready for Transformation? Determining Your Candidacy for Sexual Health Interventions

WHY FIT MEN STILL FAIL SEXUAL HEALTH TREATMENTS

Most men who walk into my practice look healthy.

They work out regularly. They watch what they eat. Their cardiovascular numbers meet all screening standards.

But their hormones tell a completely different story, one requiring restoration, not just treatment.

This is the pattern I see nearly every day. Men in reasonable physical shape, doing everything right by conventional health standards, yet hormonally bankrupt. And this disconnect explains why so many sexual health treatments fail before they even begin.

The problem starts with how we define health in the first place, and why conventional markers often miss the hormonal foundation entirely.

The Critical Importance of Proper Evaluation

Not every man is an ideal candidate for sexual health interventions, and not every intervention is right for every man. After three decades of evaluating patients, I've learned that the most successful outcomes occur when we carefully match the proper treatment to the right patient at the right time. At Biltmore Restorative Medicine & Aesthetics, our comprehensive evaluation process ensures that you're not only a suitable candidate for treatment but also that we select the optimal approach for your unique situation.

The distinction between wanting treatment and being ready for treatment is crucial. I've seen men who desperately want help but aren't prepared for the commitment required, and others who seem hesitant initially but prove to be ideal candidates once properly educated. The evaluation process helps us identify your medical suitability and readiness for the transformation journey ahead.

The Metric Most Doctors Ignore

Most physicians evaluating patients for sexual health interventions focus exclusively on medical clearance, referring to labs, cardiovascular health, and contraindications. If they check the boxes, they're cleared for treatment. But they miss the foundation entirely.

Hormone optimization isn't merely a treatment option; It's a foundational health metric. Just because your heart is healthy doesn't mean your hormones are healthy. And without optimal hormone levels, you're building on sand.

Here's what patients need to understand eating healthy, working out, and staying fit can slow the clock, but it won't stop it from ticking. Your hormones will naturally decline with age, and while lifestyle factors help, they cannot prevent the inevitable decline in gonadal hormone production.

We're outliving the lifespan of our gonadal hormone production. Unlike women who experience menopause, men face a gradual decline that can span decades.

Think of it like a tire losing air. You can have the best car, perfect maintenance, and smooth roads. But if the tire is deflating, performance suffers. Hormone restoration is akin to putting air back into a tire, rebuilding what time has depleted.

UNDERSTANDING CANDIDACY MORE THAN JUST MEDICAL CLEARANCE

Actual candidacy for sexual health treatment encompasses multiple dimensions that must all align for optimal success.

The Three Pillars of Treatment Candidacy

1. Medical Suitability

Your physical health status must be stable, with no contraindications that would prevent safe treatment. We evaluate the appropriate risk-benefit ratio for your specific situation and ensure your treatment goals are realistic and achievable.

2. Lifestyle Commitment

Your willingness to optimize health, comply with protocols, commit to long-term maintenance, and integrate healthy habits will impact treatment success.

3. Practical Readiness

Partner understanding and support, when applicable, financial planning completion, a time commitment for treatment and follow-up, and an understanding of treatment expectations ensure you can complete the journey.

Note: While emotional well-being and realistic expectations are essential factors in treatment success, Dr. Ibrahim is not a mental health specialist. Any concerns regarding psychological readiness, anxiety, depression, or relationship issues should be discussed with appropriate mental health professionals. The information provided here is for general consideration only.

The Gateway That Opens Everything Else

I recommend hormone optimization before I consider treatments like the P-Shot or acoustic wave therapy. I'll do those procedures without hormone optimization ONLY because I know it won't hurt. But that's not how I'd ever treat my brother or best friend because I feel they would be wasting their money. These procedures may help, but you'll enjoy much better results when you also optimize your hormones.

I proceed with hormone optimization alongside nearly everything else, such as smoking, alcohol use, and drug habits. We note them, but they don't stop us from beginning the foundational work.

If money is a concern, start with hormone optimization before investing in more advanced procedures. I cannot think of anything that would prevent the immediate implementation of hormone optimization.

This is the gateway to restoration. Every other intervention builds from this renewed foundation.

Comprehensive Candidacy Assessment

Cardiovascular Health

Your heart and circulatory system form the foundation of sexual function. We evaluate blood pressure control (ideally less than 140/90, preferably lower), cardiac history including previous heart attacks, strokes, or cardiac procedures, current symptoms like chest pain, shortness of breath, or exercise intolerance, medications including blood thinners, heart medications, or nitrates, and risk factors such as family history, cholesterol levels, and smoking history.

Metabolic Health

Your body's ability to process energy directly affects treatment outcomes. We assess diabetes management using HbA1c levels, ideally below 8.0%, to inform treatment considerations. However, better control (below 7.0%) optimizes outcomes, ensuring stable glucose levels without frequent swings; blood sugar control; weight status, with BMI considerations varying by treatment type; kidney function, which enables the ability to process medications and clear toxins; and liver function, which is essential for hormone metabolism.

Urological Health

As a urologist, I pay particular attention to prostate health, including PSA levels, examination findings, and family history; urinary function, noting any difficulty with urination or control; previous surgeries, including prostate procedures, hernia repairs, or other pelvic surgery; infections, considering history of urinary tract or sexually transmitted infections; and anatomical considerations, identifying any structural abnormalities.

Hormonal Status

The foundation of male sexual health includes testosterone levels (not just total, but free and bioavailable testosterone), supporting hormones (thyroid function, cortisol levels, growth factors), pituitary function (LH, FSH, and prolactin levels), estrogen balance (important for bone health and mood), and binding proteins (SHBG and other transport proteins).

Age Changes Everything About Evaluation

A 28-year-old and a 58-year-old might walk in with similar concerns, but they require fundamentally different evaluation approaches.

The younger patient needs detective work. For men under 35, I'm looking at fertility considerations first. Does he want children soon? Are his testicles functioning below par?

This is when I consider human chorionic gonadotropin (HCG). This hormone stimulates the testicles to produce both testosterone and sperm. Younger men whose gonads are still viable respond far better than older men whose testicles have passed their natural lifespan.

However, further investigation is required.

I also evaluate the pituitary gland. While rare, decreased testosterone in younger men can signal a benign pituitary adenoma. I examine Luteinizing Hormone and Follicle-Stimulating Hormone levels. If either looks suspicious, I refer them to their primary care physician for a brain MRI to rule out a pituitary mass.

The older patient needs replacement, not stimulation. We're supplementing what has naturally declined, not trying to jumpstart failing systems. This distinction matters. The wrong approach wastes time and money.

Advanced Diagnostic Testing

When I evaluate a patient, I'm not just running standard tests. At Biltmore Restorative Medicine, our evaluation goes far beyond basic lab work.

Comprehensive Laboratory Panel

- Complete Blood Count checking for anemia, infection, or blood disorders
- Comprehensive Metabolic Panel assessing liver, kidney, and electrolyte function
- Lipid Profile evaluating cholesterol, triglycerides, and cardiac risk
- Inflammatory Markers, including C-reactive protein, ESR, and other inflammation indicators
- Nutritional Assessment measuring Vitamin D, B12, folate, zinc, and magnesium levels
- Coagulation Studies evaluating bleeding and clotting function when indicated.

Specialized Testing When Indicated

- Penile Doppler Ultrasound assessing blood flow and vascular function
- Nocturnal Penile Tumescence evaluating nighttime erectile function
- Cardiac Stress Testing for men with cardiovascular risk factors
- Sleep Study if sleep apnea is suspected.

Hormone Deep Dive

Our hormone testing is the most comprehensive available, including multiple testosterone markers (total, free, bioavailable, and SHBG), estrogen metabolism (estradiol and estrone levels), thyroid complete panel (TSH, T3, T4, reverse T3, and antibodies), adrenal function (cortisol, DHEA-S, and cortisol rhythm), growth factors (IGF-1 and growth hormone assessment), and metabolic hormones (insulin, leptin, and adiponectin).

TREATMENT-SPECIFIC CANDIDACY CRITERIA

Hormone Optimization Candidacy

Ideal Candidates

In my three decades of practice, I've found the ideal candidates for hormone optimization share these characteristics: testosterone levels in the low or low-normal range, accompanied by symptoms that impact their quality of life. These symptoms typically include declining energy and motivation, mood changes like irritability or depression, sexual dysfunction including reduced libido or erectile problems, and physical changes such as muscle loss or increased body fat. Beyond the lab numbers, we look for men with stable cardiovascular health, normal prostate screening results, and a clear understanding of what testosterone optimization can and cannot achieve.

Enhanced Screening for Hormone Therapy

Additional screening may include prostate assessment, PSA, and family history; cardiovascular evaluation, including EKG, blood pressure monitoring, and lipid profile; sleep apnea screening since untreated sleep apnea is a relative contraindication; fertility considerations with sperm banking if future fertility is desired; and partner education ensuring understanding of treatment and potential effects.

Potential Exclusions

Some situations that may exclude candidates include breast cancer history since male breast cancer is hormone-sensitive, severe, untreated sleep apnea, which must be treated before hormone therapy, uncontrolled heart failure due to risk of fluid retention, and recent thromboembolic events where blood clot history requires careful evaluation.

Special Considerations

Additional considerations include age factors, where men under 35 require extra evaluation for underlying causes, athletic testing, where athletes subject to drug testing need special counseling, fertility preservation, where men who may want children need special protocols, and medication interactions, where some medications require monitoring adjustments.

P-Shot® (Priapus Shot) Candidacy

Optimal Candidates

The P-Shot® works best for men with mild to moderate erectile dysfunction (severe ED may need additional treatments), decreased sensitivity (particularly beneficial for sensation improvement), natural enhancement goals (men seeking modest improvement without surgery), Peyronie's disease in stable phase patients (not acute inflammation), and post-surgical ED after prostate surgery or other pelvic procedures.

Medical Requirements

- Normal blood clotting with no bleeding disorders or blood-thinning medications
- Absence of infections with no active urinary tract or sexually transmitted infections
- Stable health status with well-controlled chronic conditions
- Realistic anatomy with normal penile anatomy without severe deformity
- Appropriate expectations, understanding modest but meaningful improvements.

Screening Process

- Medical history focusing on bleeding disorders, infections, and medications.
- Physical examination assessing penile anatomy and circulation
- Laboratory testing, including blood counts, clotting studies, and infection screening
- Risk assessment evaluating bleeding and infection risk
- Expectation counseling with a clear discussion of realistic outcomes.

Relative Contraindications

- Active blood thinners, including Warfarin, Plavix, or other anticoagulants
- Bleeding disorders like hemophilia or other clotting problems
- Active infections, including urinary tract infections or STDs
- Unrealistic expectations, such as expecting dramatic size increases.

Priapus Toxin® Candidacy

Ideal Candidates

This treatment is perfect for men who experience significant shrinkage and identify as "growers" who want to present as "showers" even when flaccid. It's ideal for men who have body image concerns because they're bothered by their flaccid appearance in various situations. The treatment benefits men who desire a confidence boost and want improvement in their appearance in locker rooms and intimate settings. Men with premature ejaculation may also benefit since the muscle relaxation effects can help extend duration during intercourse.

Medical Requirements

Medical requirements for Priapus Toxin® include the absence of neuromuscular disorders such as myasthenia gravis or similar conditions that could be affected by botulinum toxin. You must have no known allergy to botulinum toxin, as prior reactions constitute an absolute contraindication to treatment. Your overall health status should be stable with well-controlled medical conditions that won't complicate the procedure. Realistic expectations are essential, particularly understanding the temporary nature of results and what outcomes are genuinely achievable. You must demonstrate commitment to follow-up care and show willingness to return for assessment visits and touch-up treatments as needed.

Comprehensive Screening

Comprehensive screening for Priapus Toxin® includes a neurological assessment to rule out any neuromuscular disorders that could be affected by the treatment. We take a detailed allergy history to assess prior reactions to botulinum toxin or related products. A thorough medication review identifies potential interactions with muscle relaxants or blood thinners. The anatomical evaluation assesses your specific penile anatomy and muscle function to determine optimal injection sites and expected outcomes.

Exclusions and Precautions

Several exclusions and precautions apply to Priapus Toxin® treatment. Myasthenia gravis, an autoimmune neuromuscular disorder, represents an absolute contraindication due to the risk of worsening muscle weakness. Lambert-Eaton syndrome, a rare neuromuscular condition, similarly precludes treatment with botulinum products. Active urological infections must be treated entirely before the procedure can be performed safely. Recent botulinum toxin reactions or previous adverse events to similar products make you ineligible for this treatment. Unrealistic expectations, particularly for permanent changes or dramatic size increases, indicate a need for further education, as results are temporary and improvements are modest.

Acoustic Wave Therapy Candidacy

Best Candidates

Acoustic wave therapy works optimally for vascular erectile dysfunction, meaning problems that are primarily related to blood flow restrictions. It's most effective for mild to moderate ED, though severe cases may need combination treatments with other therapies. The treatment is ideal for men seeking natural solutions who have a preference for drug-free treatments over pharmaceutical options. Preventive care candidates who want to maintain function before significant problems develop make excellent candidates. The therapy also benefits men with previous medication failures who haven't responded well to pills like Viagra or Cialis.

Health Requirements

Health requirements for acoustic wave therapy include a stable cardiovascular system with no recent history of heart attacks or unstable angina that could be exacerbated by improved blood flow. You must have no active infections, including no penile infections or open wounds in the treatment area. You cannot have penile implants since the hardware interferes with acoustic wave delivery and could potentially be damaged.

Realistic treatment expectations are essential, particularly understanding that this is a gradual improvement process rather than an immediate fix. You must demonstrate commitment to the entire series and be willing to complete the recommended 6-12 treatments for optimal results.

Medical Evaluation

A medical evaluation for acoustic wave therapy may include a cardiovascular assessment, which typically involves an EKG, blood pressure monitoring, and a detailed review of the patient's cardiac history. We perform a penile examination to assess anatomy and identify any abnormalities that might affect treatment. Infection screening rules out active infections or inflammation that could complicate therapy. We review implant history to identify prior penile surgeries or devices that might contraindicate treatment. Expectation counseling ensures a clear discussion of realistic timelines and outcomes so you understand what to expect from the treatment series.

Contraindications

Several contraindications apply to acoustic wave therapy. Active cancer in the treatment area is an absolute contraindication, as acoustic waves could theoretically spread cancer cells to other places. Bleeding disorders increase the risk of bruising or bleeding during treatment sessions. Pacemakers or defibrillators may experience electronic interference from the acoustic wave device, making treatment unsafe. Recent surgical procedures in the treatment area must fully heal before acoustic wave therapy can begin. Unrealistic expectations, particularly the expectation of immediate or dramatic results after just one or two sessions, indicate a need for further education about the gradual nature of this therapy.

What You're Actually Buying

We discuss financial considerations early in the process to ensure you're comfortable with the investment before scheduling treatment. This open conversation protects the clinical relationship and ensures we're both committed to your complete treatment journey.

However, here's what patients need to understand about stopping treatment early: it's akin to not finishing a painting. The canvas isn't ruined. There's zero harm in stopping before a planned treatment is complete.

It's not like baking a cake, where stopping midway ruins the entire process. However, stopping early won't produce the expected outcome of a complete treatment plan. You'll have something, just not what you hoped for.

The Part Your Body Must Do

I use the highest quality PRP available. The concentration and volume we achieve far exceed most practices. As a urologist, I know exactly where to place the PRP.

However, the truth is that the patient is responsible for healing and regenerating new vessels and nerves.

Some patients who are younger or healthier tend to have better responses. Patients who are diabetic, obese, or who smoke may not see excellent outcomes. More than one procedure may be necessary. These variables are beyond our control.

There is no way to predict individual response. I do not have a crystal ball, and neither does any other provider. This uncertainty makes realistic expectations critical.

LIFESTYLE AND RISK FACTOR ASSESSMENT

Modifiable Risk Factors

Cardiovascular Health Optimization

We evaluate your exercise capacity by assessing your current fitness level and exercise habits to understand your baseline cardiovascular health. Dietary patterns are reviewed to determine nutritional quality and eating habits that may affect treatment outcomes. Weight management is considered by examining BMI, body composition, and weight stability over time. Your smoking status is thoroughly reviewed, including current or previous tobacco use, since smoking significantly impacts vascular health. Alcohol consumption is evaluated by examining the pattern and quantity of alcohol use and its potential effects on sexual function and treatment success.

Sleep Quality Assessment

Sleep quality assessment includes several components. We conduct sleep apnea screening by identifying risk factors and symptoms that suggest this common, yet often undiagnosed, condition. Your sleep hygiene practices are reviewed, including bedtime routines and environmental factors that impact sleep. We evaluate sleep duration to ensure you're getting adequate sleep for optimal hormone production. Sleep quality is assessed by examining how restful your sleep feels and your energy levels upon waking.

Stress Management Evaluation

The stress management evaluation examines your work-life balance by assessing job stress levels and time management effectiveness. We discuss relaxation practices, including any exercise or other stress-relief activities you currently use. Physical activity is evaluated by examining your regular movement patterns and exercise habits in relation to stress reduction and overall health.

Note: While stress and its effects on health are important considerations, Dr. Ibrahim is not a mental health specialist. If you have concerns about stress management, anxiety, or other emotional factors affecting your health, please consult with appropriate mental health professionals.

Substance Use Assessment

Substance use assessment evaluates multiple factors. We examine alcohol's impact on sexual function and how it might affect treatment outcomes. Recreational drugs are discussed, including the use of marijuana, stimulants, or other substances that can interfere with sexual health. Your prescription medications are reviewed for their effects on sexual function and potential treatment interactions. The use of supplements is examined by reviewing over-the-counter supplements and their potential interactions with prescribed treatments. Tobacco products are assessed, including vaping, cigarettes, and smokeless tobacco, since all forms affect vascular health.

The Pattern in Who Succeeds

After evaluating thousands of men for these treatments, I've noticed a consistent pattern between transformative outcomes and modest improvements.

Patients with realistic expectations tend to have better outcomes. They also tend to be in better physical shape.

Those who are not in shape tend to blame external factors for their lack of fitness. Genetics. Their diabetes is often due to obesity. They're more sedentary, which means less cardiac capacity.

The pattern becomes apparent during the initial consultation.

If a patient presents with numerous notes from other capable physicians, I know they're unlikely to achieve great results. They're shopping for someone to fix them, not partnering in their own transformation.

I believe in self-fulfilling prophecy.

The ownership-versus-blame mindset predicts outcomes as well as any lab value. Patients who take responsibility for their health, who understand they must do the regenerative work, who come ready to restore their vitality rather than be fixed. These are the ones who experience true transformation.

FINANCIAL READINESS AND TREATMENT PLANNING

Investment Assessment

Understanding Treatment Costs

Our Initial evaluation addresses comprehensive assessment and testing costs, primary treatments, including the costs of chosen interventions, follow-up care covering ongoing monitoring and adjustment costs, maintenance needs addressing long-term treatment requirements, and potential complications, including additional expenses if problems arise.

Insurance and Payment Considerations

Most sexual health treatments aren't covered by insurance. In some cases, a procedure may be eligible for coverage through HSA/FSAs. There are other payment options, such as third-party financing and package discounts, that offer savings on comprehensive treatment approaches. It is essential to conduct a value assessment that compares the cost-benefit of quality-of-life improvement.

Financial Planning Strategies

- Budget assessment evaluating the current financial capacity for treatment
- Priority ranking determines which treatments are most important to start
- Timeline planning, spreading treatments over time if needed

- Support system, considering partner or family financial support
- Long-term planning and budgeting for maintenance and follow-up care.

AGE-SPECIFIC CONSIDERATIONS

Young Men (20-35 years)

Special Evaluation Focus

When considering treatment, take into account underlying conditions requiring more thorough investigation of sexual dysfunction causes, lifestyle factors, evaluating diet, exercise, stress, and substance use, physical health, focusing on modifiable risk factors, and financial limitations for comprehensive treatment.

Recommended Approach

Conservative treatments first start with lifestyle interventions, education emphasizing understanding normal sexual function and variation, lifestyle optimization including diet, exercise, sleep, and stress management, and careful expectation management, avoiding unrealistic enhancement goals.

Middle-Aged Men (36-55 years)

Common Presentations

Hormonal decline symptoms include beginning to experience testosterone decrease, health awareness with increased concern about aging and health, and lifestyle effects from career and family pressures affecting function.

Optimal Treatment Candidates

I find that men in this age range are ideal candidates for testosterone therapy and combination therapies using multiple treatment approaches.

They are typically ready to address lifestyle modifications and willing to invest in health-improvement and enhancement procedures.

Mature Men (55+ years)

Primary Considerations

Men in this age range often exhibit multiple health conditions with more complex medical histories, and medication interactions from multiple prescriptions affecting sexual function. They have realistic expectations, focusing on function over appearance, quality over quantity, and emphasizing sexual satisfaction over frequency, while also being concerned with partner dynamics and addressing changing relationship dynamics.

Treatment Modifications

Men in this age group require comprehensive medical clearance and a more thorough health evaluation. We often adopt a more conservative approach, using lower doses and slower progression, enhanced monitoring through more frequent follow-up and assessment, and gradual progression that takes longer to achieve optimal results, prioritizing safety over aggressive treatment.

THE BILTMORE RESTORATIVE MEDICINE EVALUATION PROCESS

Comprehensive Assessment Protocol

Step 1: Initial Consultation

An initial evaluation includes a detailed medical history with a comprehensive review of health and medications, a sexual health assessment including a thorough discussion of sexual concerns and goals, a physical examination providing a complete urological and general health examination, relationship evaluation assessing partner support when applicable, and goal setting clearly defining treatment objectives and expectations.

Step 2: Advanced Testing

Laboratory testing may include comprehensive blood work and hormone assessments, specialized studies tailored to individual presentations, and risk assessments evaluating treatment risks and contraindications.

Step 3: Results Review and Planning

Our review process includes interpreting the test results and providing a detailed explanation of all findings. We make a candidacy determination to develop a final assessment of treatment suitability, design a personalized treatment plan, and create a customized approach tailored to individual needs. We discuss the risks and benefits, provide a comprehensive review of potential outcomes, and ensure the client has a thorough understanding of the chosen treatments.

Step 4: Pre-Treatment Optimization

Health optimization involves improving modifiable risk factors by making lifestyle modifications that address diet, exercise, sleep, and stress management, adjusting medications as needed, and engaging a support system, including a partner or family as appropriate.

DECISION-MAKING FRAMEWORK

Green Light Indicators

- Clear medical candidacy with appropriate health status for chosen treatments
- Realistic expectations, understanding achievable outcomes
- Adequate support with partner and family understanding when applicable
- Financial readiness shows the ability to complete the treatment course

- Commitment to protocols demonstrating willingness to follow treatment guidelines.

Yellow Light Indicators (Proceed with Caution)

- Borderline health status that may require additional medical clearance
- Financial constraints possibly needing payment plans or phased treatment
- Lifestyle factors, including smoking, excessive drinking, or poor health habits
- Scheduling challenges with limited availability for follow-up appointments.

Red Light Indicators (Not Ready)

- Medical contraindications are health conditions that preclude treatment
- Unrealistic expectations despite counseling and education
- Financial inability where treatment would cause hardship
- Unstable health conditions, including active medical issues requiring resolution.

OPTIMIZING YOUR CANDIDACY

Health Improvement Strategies

Cardiovascular Optimization

- Regular exercise program starting with 30 minutes daily, 5 days per week
- Blood pressure control through diet, exercise, and medication compliance

- Cholesterol management using diet, exercise, and medications if needed
- Weight loss, where if BMI is over 30, aim for a 10% weight reduction
- While not required, smoking cessation is highly recommended otherwise results will not be optimal..

Hormonal Preparation

- Sleep quality improvement targeting 7-9 hours nightly with good sleep hygiene
- Stress reduction techniques using physical activity and relaxation practices
- Nutritional optimization following an anti-inflammatory diet with adequate protein
- Supplement support, including Vitamin D, zinc, magnesium, and omega-3s
- Medication review, optimizing current medications with your doctor.

Lifestyle Modifications

- Alcohol moderation, limiting alcohol to recommended guidelines
- Substance cessation, stopping recreational drugs that affect function
- Sleep optimization, improving sleep quality and duration
- Physical activity, maintaining regular exercise and movement
- Nutritional improvement, following a balanced diet supporting health goals.

THE THREE PILLARS IN PRACTICE

Medical suitability is table stakes. But it's not enough.

Hormone optimization forms the foundation. Age-appropriate evaluation ensures that we're addressing the correct issue. Financial readiness protects both patient and practice.

But the overlooked factor is psychological readiness. Your body must do the healing work. Your commitment determines whether optimization happens. Your expectations shape your perception of results.

The men who look healthy on the outside but are hormonally depleted need more than a prescription. They need a framework that addresses medical reality, lifestyle factors, and mental readiness.

Successful treatment outcomes depend on matching the right intervention to the right patient at the right time. And "right" means more than just passing a blood test.

THE DECISION PROCESS: WHEN TO PROCEED

Readiness Indicators

Proceed When

You should proceed when several indicators align. Medical clearance has been obtained with all health requirements met for your chosen treatment. Your expectations are aligned, showing a realistic understanding of likely outcomes and timelines. Support has been secured with the partner and family, as appropriate to your situation. Financial planning is complete, providing adequate resources for full treatment, including follow-up care. Your lifestyle has been optimized with health habits that support treatment success. Your commitment is demonstrated through your stated willingness to follow all protocols completely.

Wait When

You should wait until certain factors are addressed first. Health optimization is needed because modifiable risk factors are currently present, which could impair treatment success. Unrealistic expectations persist despite thorough education and counseling attempts. Major life stressors are presently affecting you, including job loss, family crisis, or significant life changes that demand your attention and resources. Financial strain exists where treatment would cause substantial hardship or require sacrificing essential needs. Unstable health conditions with active medical issues require resolution before adding treatment complexity.

Note: If you have concerns about emotional readiness, relationship factors, or other personal considerations that may impact your decision to pursue treatment, consider consulting with a qualified counselor or mental health professional. Dr. Ibrahim can provide medical guidance but is not a specialist in psychological or relationship counseling.

THE INFORMED CONSENT PROCESS

Comprehensive Education

Comprehensive education covers multiple essential topics. Treatment details include a complete explanation of all procedures and protocols you'll experience. Realistic outcomes are established through a clear discussion of expected results and timelines for improvement. Potential risks are thoroughly reviewed, including all possible complications that you should be aware of. Alternative options are discussed so you're aware of other treatment approaches that might suit your needs. Cost breakdown provides a detailed explanation of all associated costs, including follow-up and maintenance.

Decision Support

Decision support provides the framework you need to make informed choices. You have adequate time to consider options without pressure to make immediate treatment decisions. Second opinions are actively encouraged when appropriate to ensure you feel confident in your choice. Partner involvement includes significant others in discussions when desired, since sexual health affects relationships. Resource materials provide written information you can review at home and discuss with family. We welcome follow-up questions and remain available to address any questions or concerns that may arise.

CONCLUSION: YOUR READINESS ASSESSMENT

Determining candidacy for sexual health interventions requires honest self-assessment and professional medical evaluation. At Biltmore Restorative Medicine & Aesthetics, we're committed to ensuring that every patient we treat is positioned for success, both medically and practically.

Our comprehensive evaluation process may seem extensive, but it's designed to maximize your safety throughout treatment, optimize your outcomes with appropriate interventions, minimize complications through careful screening, ensure satisfaction with realistic expectations, and provide ongoing support throughout your journey.

Remember, being ready for transformation is about meeting medical criteria, optimizing your physical health, and being practically prepared for the journey ahead. The men who achieve the best results are those who approach treatment as part of a comprehensive wellness strategy, with realistic expectations and a strong commitment to success.

Key Questions for Self-Assessment

- Are my health conditions stable, well-controlled, and optimized for treatment?
- Do I have realistic expectations about treatment outcomes and timelines?
- Do I have adequate practical support (financial resources, partner understanding, time for appointments)?
- Can I commit to following all treatment protocols and lifestyle recommendations completely?
- Have I optimized my physical health through a balanced diet, regular exercise, sufficient sleep, and the elimination of harmful substances?

If you can answer "yes" to most of these questions, you may be ready to begin your transformation journey. If not, use this as a roadmap for preparation.

At Biltmore Restorative Medicine & Aesthetics, we're here to guide you through this medical evaluation process and help you determine if and when sexual health interventions are right for you from a physical health perspective. Your journey to restored vitality begins with that first conversation, and we're committed to helping you rebuild optimal function and ensuring you're medically prepared for success.

Important Disclaimer: While this chapter addresses various aspects of treatment readiness, Dr. Ibrahim is a specialist in men's sexual health and urology, not in mental health, psychology, or relationship counseling. Any concerns regarding emotional well-being, stress management, anxiety, depression, relationship dynamics, or other psychological factors should be discussed with appropriate mental health professionals. The information provided here regarding these topics is for general consideration only and does not constitute a psychological evaluation or counseling.

References

Fode M, Hatzichristodoulou G, Serefoglu EC, et al.
Low-intensity shockwave therapy for erectile dysfunction: is the evidence strong enough?
Nat Rev Urol. 2017;14(10)593-606.
PMID 28741629
https//pubmed.ncbi.nlm.nih.gov/28741629/

Lu Z, Lin G, Reed-Maldonado A, et al.
Effects of Low-Intensity Extracorporeal Shockwave Therapy on Erectile Dysfunction A Systematic Review and Meta-Analysis.
Urology. 2017;99107-116.
PMID 27986492
https//pubmed.ncbi.nlm.nih.gov/27986492/

Appel B, Kitrey N, Wernovsky G, et al.
Low Intensity Shock Wave Treatment for Erectile Dysfunction-How Long Does the Effect Last?
J Urol. 2018;199(4)1111-1115.
PMID 29477719
https//pubmed.ncbi.nlm.nih.gov/29477719/

Hayon S, Panken EJ, Bennett NE.
Variations in Low Intensity Shockwave Treatment Protocols for Erectile Dysfunction.
World J Mens Health. 2024;42(2)283-289.
PMID 37853533
https//pubmed.ncbi.nlm.nih.gov/37853533/

CHAPTER 5

The Revolution in Non-Surgical Enhancement: Cutting-Edge Treatments That Actually Work

YOU'RE NOT DEFICIENT IN VIAGRA.

Penile implants are the last resort.

Yet somehow, they've become the first conversation for too many men struggling with sexual function. I've watched this pattern for three decades as a urologist trained at Duke. Men come in expecting surgery. Their previous doctors told them it's the gold standard.

It's not the first option.

Surgery is what you do when everything else has failed. But here's what most men don't know: hundreds of my patients were told they needed surgery, gave the Priapus shot and hormone optimization a try instead, and achieved exactly what they wanted.

In clinical studies, over 85% reported erections that satisfied both themselves and their partners. That's a lot of men saved from a permanent surgical procedure with none of the risks.

THE DAWN OF A NEW ERA IN MALE SEXUAL HEALTH.

As a Duke University-trained urologist who has witnessed the evolution of male sexual health treatment over three decades, I can confidently say we're living in the most exciting time in the history of sexual medicine. The combination of regenerative medicine, advanced biotechnology, and precision medical techniques has created treatment options that were pure science fiction when I began practicing.

At Biltmore Restorative Medicine & Aesthetics, we've been at the forefront of implementing these revolutionary treatments. Unlike franchise clinics that offer cookie-cutter approaches, our independent practice allows us to customize cutting-edge therapies to each patient's unique needs and goals.

The transformation in male sexual health treatment has been nothing short of remarkable. When I started practicing urology in the early 1990s, our options were limited to basic medications, primitive devices, or high-risk surgeries. Today, we have sophisticated, scientifically backed treatments that can address not just symptoms, but actually regenerate and restore sexual function at a cellular level.

THE REGENERATION YOUR BODY ALREADY KNOWS HOW TO DO

Remember your peak years? Many men experienced easy, frequent performance without difficulty.

Viagra wasn't even invented yet.

Today, at age 60, you're not deficient in Viagra. You're most likely lacking in testosterone. And your blood vessels aren't as young and spry as they were at 25. You need to refresh the blood and nerve supply.

That regeneration is what the P-Shot does at the cellular level.

When I inject platelet-rich plasma into penile tissue, it stimulates the formation of more blood vessels and nerves. An erection needs both neurological and vascular input. The P-Shot promotes both of these formations.

You're not managing symptoms. You're regenerating tissue.

The science is straightforward. Platelet-rich plasma (PRP) contains growth factors that signal your body to build new infrastructure. More vessels mean more blood flow. More nerves mean better sensitivity. Both together mean function returns.

But PRP alone isn't the complete picture.

WHY NON-SURGICAL SOLUTIONS HAVE BECOME THE GOLD STANDARD.

The Paradigm Shift.

The move toward non-surgical treatments represents a fundamental shift in how we approach male sexual health.

From Symptom Management to Root Cause Treatment

Traditional approaches focused on masking symptoms, but they didn't address the underlying causes. Modern treatments address the underlying physiological problems that create dysfunction in the first place. Regenerative medicine actually heals and restores tissues rather than just covering up the issue. These approaches provide long-term solutions rather than temporary fixes that require constant maintenance.

From One-Size-Fits-All to Personalized Medicine

Customized protocols are replacing the generic treatments that dominated medicine for decades. Individual patient factors now guide treatment selection, rather than adhering to rigid protocols. Combination therapies are tailored to meet specific needs rather than offering a one-size-fits-all approach. Ongoing adjustments based on response and results allow us to optimize outcomes for each patient.

Comprehensive Advantages of Non-Surgical Approaches.

Superior Safety Profile

The treatment carries a minimal risk of serious complications, with infection rates under 1%. No general anesthesia is required, which means we're avoiding the surgical and anesthetic risks that come with operating rooms. Lower infection rates result from office-based procedures that employ sterile techniques, eliminating the exposure risks associated with hospitals. Reduced scarring potential results from minimally invasive approaches that don't require large incisions or tissue destruction.

Enhanced Effectiveness

Results are comparable to or better than those of surgery, without any of the associated risks. More natural-looking outcomes are possible because we're focused on enhancement rather than reconstruction. Gradual, progressive improvement allows the body to adapt over time rather than shocking the system with sudden change. The treatments are reversible if desired and can be adjusted or modified as your needs change. Customization to individual anatomy ensures results that look natural on your specific body rather than following a generic template.

Practical Convenience

Office-based procedures require no hospital stays or surgical centers. The treatment offers minimal downtime with return to work and activities within hours rather than weeks. We provide same-day treatment with most procedures completed in a single visit. No hospitalization is required, which eliminates hospital costs and complications.

Economic Advantages

Lower overall costs make these treatments significantly less expensive than surgical alternatives. No hospital fees means we're eliminating facility and anesthesia charges that can add thousands to your bill. The therapy offers reduced recovery expenses because there's no time off work or need for recovery assistance. We provide payment plan options with flexible financing that make treatment accessible without financial strain.

WHY I LAYER TREATMENTS INSTEAD OF CHOOSING ONLY ONE.

Think of it this way, why turn on the sprinklers if the fire is in a waste basket?

We're treating the area of need directly, not flooding your whole system with a foreign substance like Viagra. We're going straight to the source.

That's where acoustic wave therapy comes in. These treatments create what we call iatrogenic injuries. Controlled micro-trauma signals the PRP and human cellular tissue products to rush to the area.

They deliver growth factors that promote the growth of blood vessels and nerves. More blood. More sensitivity.

The acoustic waves and the PRP compound upon each other. One creates the call for help. The approach includes the other answers with regenerative power.

Add testosterone optimization to this combination, and you're addressing both desire and mechanical function simultaneously.

The P-Shot won't stimulate libido at all—hormones and the P-Shot address different areas. Testosterone increases desire and acts as a vasodilator, increasing blood flow. The P-Shot increases blood flow and nerve function.

They work on different timelines as well. Hormones work quickly, often within days. The P-Shot can take up to two months for enough new vessels and nerves to form.

But the wait is worth it.

Patients who choose just one modality tend to have a 75% satisfaction rate. Most report moderate to high satisfaction. But combination patients? Well above 90% report complete satisfaction.

That jump from 75% to over 90% isn't marginal. It's the difference between "pretty good" and "exactly what I wanted.".

ADVANCED PRP THERAPY: THE P-SHOT® EVOLUTION

Beyond Basic PRP: Our Advanced Protocol

While many providers offer basic PRP treatments, our advanced P-Shot® protocol represents the evolution of platelet-rich plasma therapy.

Enhanced Concentration Techniques

Double-spin processing yields higher platelet concentrations compared to standard techniques. Growth factor activation optimizes the release of healing factors before injection. Quality assurance testing ensures optimal platelet counts, allowing us to deliver precisely what we promise. Customized preparation adjusts the protocol based on individual characteristics, such as age and health status.

Precision Injection Methodology

Anatomical mapping uses ultrasound guidance when appropriate to identify optimal injection sites. Multiple injection sites optimize coverage and distribution throughout the tissue. Depth variation targets different tissue layers for comprehensive treatment. Our protocol includes volume optimization, with precise amounts calculated to ensure maximum effectiveness.

Combination Enhancement

Acoustic wave pre-treatment prepares tissues for optimal PRP absorption before the procedure. Nutritional optimization ensures your body has the building blocks it needs for optimal healing. Our protocol includes hormone coordination, which optimizes treatment timing based on hormone levels. We address lifestyle synchronization that coordinates with the patient's health optimization efforts to ensure the best results.

THE SCIENCE BEHIND ADVANCED PRP.

Growth Factor Profiles

Modern PRP analysis reveals over 30 different growth factors

- PDGF (Platelet-Derived Growth Factor) stimulates cell division and angiogenesis.
- VEGF (Vascular Endothelial Growth Factor) promotes the formation of new blood vessels.
- EGF (Epidermal Growth Factor) enhances tissue healing and regeneration.
- FGF (Fibroblast Growth Factor) supports tissue repair and growth.
- TGF-β (Transforming Growth Factor) regulates cell growth and differentiation.

Mechanisms of Action

This process involves angiogenesis, the formation of new blood vessels that improve circulation. The approach encompasses neurogenesis, which enhances sensitivity, and tissue regeneration, facilitating the healing and renewal of damaged tissues. Inflammatory modulation reduces chronic inflammation that impairs function.

Enhanced P-Shot® Outcomes.

Functional Improvements

Patients using our advanced protocol typically experience an enhancement in erectile quality, with 75-85% of patients reporting significant improvement. 85-95% of patients experience sensitivity restoration. Results include improved performance over longer durations, with increased stamina and endurance, and a return to natural response with the return of spontaneous erectile function.

Physical Enhancement

Results include appearance improvement with enhanced flaccid and erect appearance. Patients achieve texture enhancement with improved skin quality and sensitivity, while proportion optimization maintains natural-looking results.

Timeline and Duration

Patients typically experience initial improvement, with noticeable changes occurring within 2-4 weeks. The approach includes significant enhancement with major improvements at 6-8 weeks. Patients typically achieve their peak results and maximum benefits within 3-6 months. Results include duration with benefits normally lasting 12-18 months.

Patient Success Story

"The advanced P-Shot® protocol at Biltmore exceeded every expectation I had. Not only did my erectile function improve dramatically, but the sensitivity enhancement has revolutionized my intimate life. At 52, I'm performing better than I did in my twenties. The natural approach gave me confidence that I made the right choice."

–Michael, age 52

THE MARRIAGE I DIDN'T KNOW I WAS SAVING.

I had a patient whose wife was planning to leave him.

He came in for sexual function issues. After a standard consultation, we started him on hormone optimization and performed the Priapus shot.

Two months later, he told me his marriage was saved.

His mood improved so much. His sexual abilities improved so much. Their relationship improved more than it had in years.

I wasn't just treating erectile function. I was working on a man's confidence, his sense of self, and his connection to his partner. When you address the root physiological issues, everything downstream improves.

Sexual health isn't isolated. It touches everything.

Your relationships. Your confidence. Your willingness to be intimate. Your partner's satisfaction and security. The psychological weight of feeling like you've lost something fundamental to your identity as a man.

Pills can't give you that back. Surgery is irreversible. But regeneration? Regeneration restores what was naturally yours.

NEXT-GENERATION ACOUSTIC WAVE THERAPY.

Beyond Standard Shockwave Treatment.

Advanced Technology Features

Focused shockwaves provide precise energy delivery to target tissues. Variable-frequency settings are customized to individual anatomy, and real-time monitoring ensures that optimal treatment parameters are maintained. The approach includes computer-controlled delivery, which provides consistent and precise energy application.

Treatment Protocol Optimization

Patients experience individualized parameters with progressive intensity, delivering a gradual increase. Anatomical targeting focuses on specific areas based on individual needs. The treatment often involves coordinating a combination of procedures to maximize effect.

The Comprehensive Acoustic Wave Therapy Experience.

Pre-Treatment Preparation

- Vascular assessment evaluates blood flow and circulation
- Treatment planning customizes the protocol based on individual anatomy.
- Baseline measurements document current function for comparison.
- Health optimization ensures optimal conditions for treatment response.
- Education helps patients understand the treatment process and what to expect.

Treatment Sessions

- Comfortable positioning in a relaxed environment ensures optimal treatment.
- The approach includes precise application with computer-controlled energy delivery.
- Patients experience real-time monitoring with continuous assessment of treatment response.
- Comfort management ensures patient comfort throughout the procedure.

Post-Treatment Optimization

- Activity recommendations provide specific guidelines for optimal healing.

- Lifestyle support continues health optimization practices.
- Patients experience progress monitoring with regular assessment of improvement.
- Protocol adjustments modify treatment based on response.
- Maintenance planning involves long-term care strategies.

Advanced Acoustic Wave Therapy Results.

Vascular Improvements

Acoustic wave therapy promotes the formation of new blood vessels, resulting in a measurable increase in penile blood flow. Existing vessel enhancement improves the function of the current circulation, and micro-plaque removal clears blockages in small blood vessels. Endothelial function improves blood vessel wall function.

Functional Enhancements

- Patients experience erectile firmness with 70-80% of patients reporting significantly harder erections.
- Results include improved duration and enhanced ability to maintain erections.
- Patients achieve recovery time with shorter refractory periods between sexual encounters.
- Patients gain spontaneous function with a return to natural erectile response.

Performance Benefits

- Patients experience enhanced sensitivity, improved nerve function, and increased sensation.
- The therapy improves response time with faster arousal and erectile response.
- Enhanced endurance for sexual stamina and performance.

- Confidence brings dramatic psychological benefits.
- Partner satisfaction and intimate relationships are improved.

Long-Term Outcomes

- Sustained improvement with benefits lasting several months.
- Progressive enhancement with continued improvement over time.
- Maintenance protocols maintain benefits with treatments every 3 months.
- Improvement in overall quality of life with enhanced sexual satisfaction.

THE PILL THAT ISN'T SOLVING YOUR REAL PROBLEM

Most men have been conditioned to think a pill is the easiest solution.

Take Viagra. Wait 30 minutes. Hope it works. Deal with the side effects. Repeat as often as you want to be intimate.

But Viagra doesn't fix anything. It temporarily overrides a system that's declining. You're still deficient in testosterone. Your blood vessels are still aging. Your nerve supply is still diminishing.

The pill is a band-aid on a wound that needs stitches.

What I offer is different. I'm treating the area of need directly, building new blood vessels and growing new nerves, and optimizing the hormones that make desire possible in the first place.

This is why my proprietary techniques, such as Priapus Toxin and RestoreMore, exist. To address the specific gaps that pills and generic treatments miss.

I'm not flooding the whole house with water. I'm putting out the fire in the waste basket.

REVOLUTIONARY ENHANCEMENT TECHNOLOGIES

Priapus Toxin® Precision Neuromodulation

This breakthrough treatment addresses one of men's most common concerns with unprecedented precision.

Advanced Injection Techniques

- Micro-needle technology minimizes discomfort and tissue trauma.
- The procedure includes anatomical mapping with precise identification of target muscle groups.
- Multi-zone treatment provides comprehensive coverage for optimal results.
- Depth variation targets different tissue layers.

Customized Treatment Protocols

- Individual assessment tailors treatment to specific anatomy.
- A goal-oriented approach tailors the procedure to desired outcomes.
- Progressive treatment builds results over multiple sessions.
- Maintenance scheduling optimizes long-term results.

Enhanced Results

- Flaccid enhancement with 15-30% improvement in non-erect appearance.
- Patients experience a confidence boost, accompanied by a dramatic improvement in self-perception.
- Functional benefits include enhanced erectile quality and control.
- Natural appearance maintains proportional enhancement.
- Improved partner satisfaction during intimate experiences.

Patient Experience

"The Priapus Toxin® treatment was a game-changer for my confidence. Not only do I look better in every situation, but my overall sexual function has improved as well. The procedure was quick and comfortable, and the results have exceeded my expectations."

–David, age 39

RESTOREMORE ADVANCED GIRTH ENHANCEMENT

Our proprietary girth enhancement protocol represents the pinnacle of non-surgical enhancement.

Advanced Filler Technology

- Next-generation materials use the latest FDA-approved enhancement products.
- Biocompatible integration with materials that integrate naturally with tissue.
- Reversible options can be adjusted or removed if desired.
- Longevity optimization for enhanced duration of results.

Precision Injection Techniques

- 3D anatomical modeling helps us understand the individual architecture of the penis.
- Multi-layer approach targets different tissue depths.
- Symmetry optimization ensures balanced, natural enhancement.
- Texture preservation maintains natural feel and function.
- Safety protocols with comprehensive risk management.

RestoreMore Advantages

- Patients experience natural integration with seamless incorporation into existing tissues.
- Proportional enhancement maintains aesthetic balance.
- Functional preservation with no interference with sexual function.
- Customizable results are adjustable to individual goals.
- Reversibility allows modifications if needed.

Expected Outcomes

- Girth increases by 25-45% in circumference.
- An increase in circumference from 4.5" to 6" is a104% increase in volume.
- A natural feel with a soft, natural texture is maintained.
- Immediate results with enhancement visible right after treatment.
- Typical duration of 12-18 months.

WHAT'S COMING NEXT IN MALE SEXUAL HEALTH?

I've been using regenerative approaches for nearly a decade. These products have been available in the USA for about nine or ten years.

That experience has shown me where we're headed.

Human cellular tissue products will become more and more common in the years to come. Umbilical and placental HCTPs contain billions, if not trillions, more growth factors than PRP.

The results I'm seeing with these advanced treatments are remarkable. But there's a massive gap between what's scientifically possible and what's institutionally accepted.

The FDA considers these products experimental. Many malpractice carriers won't insure their use. So providers are hesitant, even when they see the potential.

What's holding us back isn't the science. It's mainly due to the lack of acceptance by the medical community and liability insurance companies.

But that's changing. Slowly. As more men experience life-changing results without surgery, the pressure builds. The evidence accumulates. The old guard has to acknowledge what's working.

In five to ten years, regenerative approaches will be standard first-line treatment. Surgery will return to its proper place as the last resort, not the first conversation.

TREATMENT COMBINATIONS: SYNERGISTIC ENHANCEMENT

The Complete Enhancement Protocol

Combining multiple treatments can create synergistic effects that exceed the effects of individual therapies.

Phase 1 Preparation and Foundation (Weeks 1-4)

- Health optimization maximizes baseline health status.
- Hormone evaluation ensures an optimal hormonal environment.
- Lifestyle modification implements supportive health practices.
- Baseline assessment documents current function and appearance.

Phase 2 Regenerative Enhancement (Weeks 5-12)

- The Advanced P-Shot stimulates tissue regeneration and growth.

- The Acoustic Wave Therapy Series optimizes vascular function and blood flow.
- Patients experience progress monitoring with regular assessment of improvement.
- A protocol adjustment modifies treatment based on the response.

Phase 3 Targeted Enhancement (Weeks 13-20)

- Priapus Toxin® optimizes appearance and function.
- RestoreMore for girth enhancement if desired.
- Final optimization fine-tunes all aspects of enhancement.

Phase 4 Maintenance and Optimization (Ongoing)

- Regular monitoring with quarterly assessments and adjustments.
- Touch-up treatments maintain optimal results.
- Lifestyle support continues health optimization practices.
- Long-term planning allows for adjustments to treatment as needs evolve.

TECHNOLOGY INTEGRATION AND INNOVATION

Precision Diagnostics

Advanced Assessment Tools

- Penile Doppler ultrasound measures blood flow and vascular function.
- Nocturnal tumescence monitoring assesses natural erectile function.
- Sensitivity testing evaluates nerve function and response.
- 3D imaging for anatomical mapping helps with treatment planning.

- Performance metrics provide an objective measure of improvement.

Real-Time Monitoring

- Response tracking with immediate assessment of intervention effects.
- Safety monitoring with continuous evaluation of patient well-being.
- Protocol optimization with real-time adjustments for optimal outcomes.
- Data collection that provides comprehensive treatment records.

Artificial Intelligence Integration

Treatment Optimization

- Protocol customization with AI-assisted treatment planning.
- This works by predicting outcomes using predictive modeling to assess treatment success.
- Risk assessment with advanced analysis of complication risks.
- Response optimization that tailors treatments to individual characteristics.

Patient Monitoring

- Progress tracking with continuous assessment of improvement patterns.
- Early intervention identifies issues before they become problems.
- Outcome enhancement optimizes protocols based on response data.
- Long-term planning supports sustained results.

COMPARING TREATMENT MODALITIES

Effectiveness Comparison.

Single Treatment Outcomes

- P-Shot® alone 70-80% satisfaction, moderate enhancement.
- Acoustic Wave Therapy alone 65-75% satisfaction, functional improvement focus.
- Priapus Toxin® alone 80-90% satisfaction, appearance enhancement.
- RestoreMore alone 85-95% satisfaction, girth enhancement.

Combination Treatment Outcomes

- P-Shot® + Acoustic Wave Therapy 85-90% satisfaction, comprehensive functional improvement.
- P-Shot® + Priapus Toxin® 90-95% satisfaction, function, and appearance enhancement.
- Complete protocol 95-98% satisfaction, comprehensive transformation.

Long-Term Success Rates

- Patients using comprehensive protocols for over 12 months report satisfaction rates of 90-95%.
- Over 24 months, with proper maintenance, we see an 85-90% satisfaction rate and a
- 36-month satisfaction rate of 80-85% with ongoing optimization. 95% of patients report an improvement in their quality of life and overall satisfaction.

Safety Profile Comparison

Complication Rates

- P-Shot® <1% serious complications, 5-10% minor side effects.
- Acoustic Wave Therapy has <0.5% complications and minimal side effects.
- Priapus Toxin® <2% complications, 10-15% minor side effects.
- RestoreMore <3% serious complications, 15-20% minor side effects.

Risk Mitigation

- Comprehensive screening identifies and manages risk factors.
- Expert techniques by experienced providers reduce complication rates.
- Quality materials involve the use of only FDA-approved products and devices.
- Follow-up care with immediate attention to any concerns or complications.

PATIENT SELECTION FOR ADVANCED TREATMENTS.

Optimal Candidates

Physical Criteria

- Good general health, stable medical conditions, and routine healing.
- Realistic anatomy with standard penile structure and function.
- Stable relationships with a supportive partner or a comfortable single status.
- Financial readiness with the ability to invest in comprehensive treatment.

Psychological Readiness

- Realistic expectations with understanding of achievable outcomes.
- Internal motivation with personal desire for improvement.
- Emotional stability with the ability to handle the treatment process.
- Open communication with the client to discuss any concerns.

Treatment-Specific Considerations

- P-Shot® candidates are men with mild-moderate ED or sensitivity issues.
- Acoustic Wave Therapy candidates have vascular ED or desire drug-free solutions.
- Priapus Toxin® candidates have concerns about appearance or shrinkage.
- RestoreMore candidates have girth-enhancement goals or body-image concerns.

Exclusion Criteria

Medical Contraindications

- Active cancer in the treatment area or requiring active therapy.
- Severe cardiovascular disease, including unstable angina or a recent heart attack.
- Bleeding disorders affect blood clotting - active infections, local or systemic.
- Autoimmune disorders can affect the healing process or immune function.

Psychological Contraindications

- Unrealistic expectations persist despite extensive counseling.
- Body dysmorphic disorder with excessive preoccupation with appearance.
- Severe depression with untreated major depressive disorder.
- Relationship instability with active marital conflict or relationship problems.

MAXIMIZING TREATMENT OUTCOMES

Pre-Treatment Optimization

Health Maximization

- Cardiovascular fitness with regular exercise and heart health optimization.
- Nutritional status with an anti-inflammatory diet and nutritional supplementation.
- Hormonal balance through testosterone optimization when appropriate.
- Sleep quality ensures adequate rest for healing and recovery.

Lifestyle Preparation

- Smoking cessation with complete tobacco cessation at least 4 weeks prior. Results for smokers will not be optimal.
- Alcohol moderation limits alcohol consumption before and after treatment.
- Supplement optimization adds nutrients that support the body's natural healing process.
- An exercise routine establishes a regular physical activity routine.
- Relationship preparation includes discussing treatment with partners.

Post-Treatment Care.

Immediate Care (First 48 hours)

- Activity modification, avoiding strenuous physical activity.
- Hygiene protocols follow specific cleaning instructions.
- Medication compliance, taking prescribed medications as directed.
- Monitoring for any signs of complications.
- Communication and staying in contact with our office.

Short-Term Care (First 2 weeks)

- Gradual increase in activities, returning to normal.
- Sexual activity timing follows guidelines for resuming intimacy.
- Follow-up appointments for progress assessments.
- Lifestyle maintenance to continue healthy habits.
- Report concerns promptly to address any issues.

Long-Term Optimization (Ongoing)

- Lifestyle maintenance to continue health optimization practices.
- Regular monitoring with scheduled follow-up appointments.
- Touch-up treatments to maintain results.
- Health evolution to adapt care as health status changes.
- Nurturing a relationship to maintain an intimate connection.

HOW TO CHOOSE A PROVIDER WHO ACTUALLY KNOWS WHAT THEY'RE DOING.

Experience is the main thing.

A decade of hands-on experience with these protocols provides you with pattern recognition that newer providers simply don't have. You learn which combinations work best for which patients. You understand the timelines. You can manage expectations realistically.

Too many providers are jumping on trends without the depth of knowledge to deliver consistent results. They make unrealistic promises. They don't understand the science. They haven't treated hundreds of patients through the full regeneration cycle.

Ask how long they've been using these treatments. Ask about their training. Ask about their outcomes.

If they're promising overnight miracles, walk away. If they can't explain cellular mechanisms clearly, walk away. If they don't discuss combination protocols, walk away.

Real expertise is specific. It's measured. It's honest about timelines and realistic about outcomes.

The right provider will tell you that hormones work quickly, but the P-Shot takes two months. They'll explain why acoustic wave therapy amplifies PRP. They'll discuss the difference between 75% and 90% satisfaction rates with combination approaches.

They'll also tell you the truth.   I wish every man understood before jumping to surgery.

FINANCIAL INVESTMENT AND VALUE

Treatment Investment Analysis

Individual Treatment Costs:	
Advanced P-Shot®	$2,000-2,500 per treatment.
Acoustic Wave Therapy series	$4,000- $ 6,000 for the complete protocol.
Priapus Toxin®	$1,500-2,200 per treatment.
RestoreMore	$5,000-10,000 depending on goals.

Comprehensive Protocol Investment

Complete enhancement program	$12,000-20,000.
Package discounts	15-25% savings for comprehensive treatment.
Financing options	12-60 month payment plans available.

Return on Investment

- Quality of life improvement with immeasurable enhancement in life satisfaction.
- Relationship benefits include improved intimacy and partner satisfaction.

- Patients experience a professional and personal confidence boost.
- Health benefits with overall wellness improvements.
- Long-term value offers sustained benefits over time.

COMPARISON TO ALTERNATIVES:

Vs. Surgical Options:

- Cost 40-60% less than surgical alternatives.
- Safety Significantly lower complication rates.
- Recovery Days instead of months.
- Results Comparable or superior outcomes.
- Reversibility Can be adjusted or modified.

Vs. Medication Management:

- **Annual cost:** Often less than long-term medication expenses.
- **Effectiveness:** Addresses root causes rather than symptoms.
- **Side effects:** Minimal compared to those of the drugs.
- **Convenience:** No daily medication requirements.
- **Spontaneity:** No timing restrictions for sexual activity.

CHOOSING THE RIGHT PROVIDER

Critical Selection Factors

Medical Qualifications

- Expertise with relevant specialty training, with urology preferred.

- Experience level with hundreds or thousands of procedures performed.
- Training credentials with formal training in sexual medicine.
- Research involvement that contributes to scientific advancement.
- Ongoing education demonstrates commitment to staying current.

Facility Standards

- Proper medical facility licensing and accreditation.
- State-of-the-art devices and technology ensure the highest quality of equipment.
- Safety protocols with comprehensive infection control and emergency procedures.
- Support staff includes qualified nurses and medical assistants.

Treatment Approach

- Comprehensive evaluation with thorough assessment and treatment planning.
- Customized protocols provide individualized rather than cookie-cutter approaches.
- Multiple options offer various treatment modalities.
- Realistic expectations through honest discussion of achievable outcomes.
- Follow-up care ensures long-term support and optimization.

RED FLAGS TO AVOID

Provider Concerns

- Unrealistic promises guarantee specific outcomes or dramatic results.
- High-pressure sales tactics often prompt immediate decisions or limited-time offers.
- Unqualified staff with non-physicians performing medical procedures.
- Limited experience with providers new to sexual medicine.
- Poor communication indicates an inability to explain treatments clearly.

Facility Issues

- An unlicensed operation operates without proper medical facility licensing.
- Poor hygiene with unclean facilities or inadequate sterilization.
- Emergency preparedness is lacking, with no protocols in place for handling complications.
- Privacy concerns show inadequate confidentiality protections.

THE BILTMORE RESTORATIVE MEDICINE ADVANTAGE

Why Choose Biltmore Restorative Medicine?

Unique Qualifications

- Dr. George K. Ibrahim is a urologist with 30+ years of experience.
- He has Duke University training with an academic medical center background.

- He has earned expertise in sexual medicine through specialized training and certification.

Comprehensive Approach

- As an independent practice, we're not a franchise operation with corporate limitations.
- We offer customized care with individualized treatment protocols for each patient.
- We invest in advanced technology using the latest equipment and most effective techniques.
- We offer ongoing support with long-term care relationships.

Patient-Centered Care

- Detailed consultations provide comprehensive evaluation and treatment planning.
- Realistic expectations through honest assessment of achievable outcomes.
- Quality assurance maintains the highest standards for safety and effectiveness.
- Accessible support is available throughout treatment and beyond.

Our Commitment to Excellence

Clinical Excellence

- Advanced training through continuous education in the latest techniques.
- Achieve quality outcomes with superior results that surpass industry standards.
- Our safety record demonstrates an exceptional safety profile with minimal complications.

- Patient satisfaction is consistently high.

Innovation Leadership

- Treatment advancement develops and refines protocols.
- Adopting technology through early adoption of proven innovations.
- Research participation contributes to scientific advancement.
- Education provision trains other providers in advanced techniques.
- Protocol development creates new treatment approaches.

You Don't Have To Accept The Last Resort First

Thousands of men have safely avoided surgery with these regenerative approaches.

They've restored the function they desired. They've saved their relationships. They've restored confidence they thought was gone forever.

All without the risks of a permanent surgical procedure.

You're not deficient in Viagra. You're not destined for implants. You're a candidate for regeneration if you choose a provider who understands how to orchestrate these treatments properly.

The body wants to heal itself. It requires the right inputs at the right time, in the right combination.

- Blood vessels.
- Nerves.
- Hormones.
- Growth factors.
- Acoustic stimulation.
- Time.

That's the formula that's worked for hundreds of my patients. That's what 85% to 90% satisfaction looks like in practice. That's what saved a marriage I didn't even know was at risk.

Surgery is still there if you need it. But you probably don't.

Not yet. Not if you try regeneration first.

Real Patient Transformations

"The comprehensive non-surgical program at Biltmore completely transformed my life. The combination of P-Shot®, Acoustic Wave Therapy, and Priapus Toxin® gave me results I never thought possible without surgery. At 55, I'm more confident and satisfied than I've been in decades."

—Robert, age 55

"After researching all my options, I chose Biltmore because of Dr. Ibrahim's expertise and the comprehensive approach. The results exceeded my expectations, and the care was exceptional throughout the entire process." -

—James, age 42

"I was skeptical about non-surgical treatments, but the science convinced me to try. The combination therapy approach gave me dramatic improvements in both function and appearance. I wish I had done this years ago."

—Michael, age 48

YOUR NEXT STEPS

The revolution in non-surgical male enhancement has created unprecedented opportunities for men to restore their sexual vitality and confidence safely and effectively.

At Biltmore Restorative Medicine & Aesthetics, we're committed to helping you navigate these options and choose the treatments that best match your goals, health status, and lifestyle. Our comprehensive approach ensures that you receive not only advanced treatments but also the education, support, and ongoing care necessary for optimal results.

Key Takeaways

- Non-surgical treatments are now the gold standard for male sexual enhancement.
- Combination protocols produce superior results compared to single treatments.
- Advanced techniques and technologies are delivering unprecedented outcomes.
- Safety profiles are excellent when performed by qualified providers.
- Results are sustainable with proper maintenance and follow-up care.
- Provider selection is crucial for optimal outcomes and safety.

The question isn't whether these treatments work; the evidence is clear and the results speak for themselves. The question is whether you're ready to take advantage of these advances to transform your sexual health and overall quality of life.

Your journey to renewed vitality begins with a single conversation. Contact Biltmore Restorative Medicine & Aesthetics today to learn how these revolutionary treatments can help you feel like the best version of yourself again.

We can't wait to help you feel like YOU again!.

References

Symonds T, Perelman MA, Althof S, et al.
Development and validation of a premature ejaculation diagnostic tool.
Eur Urol. 2007;52(2)565-573.
PMID 17275165
https//pubmed.ncbi.nlm.nih.gov/17275165/

CHAPTER 6

Natural Optimization Strategies: Lifestyle Changes That Make a Real Difference

YOU'RE NOT VIAGRA DEFICIENT, YOU'RE TESTOSTERONE DEFICIENT

After thirty years in practice, I continue to correct the same misconception.

Men in their fifties, sixties, and beyond walk into my office expecting to perform as they did at twenty-five. They want the magic pill they saw on TV.

Here's what I tell them: When you were in your twenties, and you could perform multiple times nightly, Viagra hadn't been invented yet.

You weren't Viagra deficient then. You're not Viagra deficient now.

You're testosterone-deficient.

The Decline Starts Earlier Than You Think

Testosterone levels typically begin their gradual decline around age twenty-two. Not forty. Not fifty. Twenty-two.

It's downhill from there.

By the time a man reaches his sixties, his testosterone is roughly one-third of what it was at peak. The math is simple: you can't expect peak performance with a third of the fuel.

Yet somehow, we've convinced an entire generation of men that a pill will solve what's fundamentally a hormone problem.

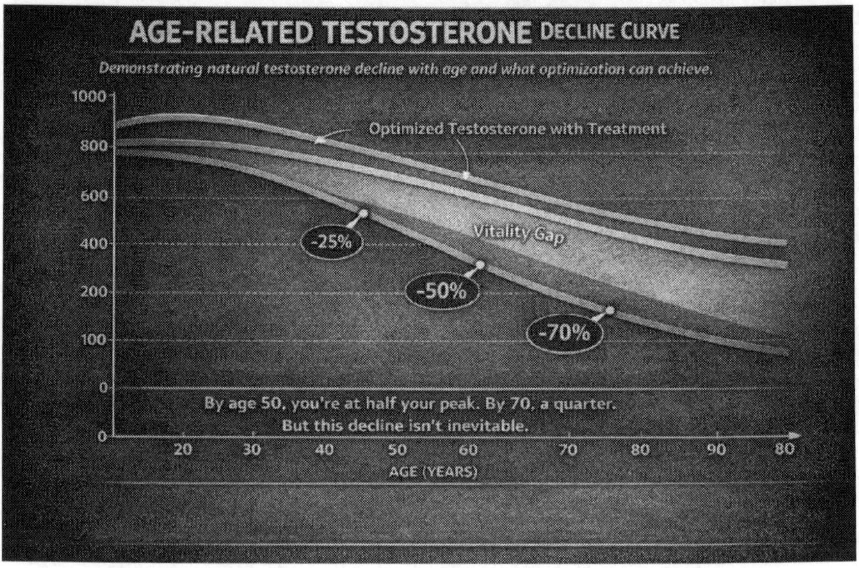

THE FOUNDATION OF SEXUAL HEALTH: MORE THAN JUST TREATMENT

While advanced medical treatments can produce remarkable results, they are most effective when built upon a foundation of optimal health and wellness. After thirty years of treating men's sexual health issues, I've learned that the most successful patients are those who approach their sexual wellness holistically, combining cutting-edge treatments with proven lifestyle optimization strategies.

At Biltmore Restorative Medicine & Aesthetics, we don't just treat symptoms... we help men transform their entire approach to health and vitality. This chapter will provide you with the same evidence-based lifestyle strategies we recommend to our patients, strategies that can dramatically enhance the effectiveness of any medical treatment while providing benefits that extend far beyond the bedroom.

Why the Disconnect Exists

Pharmaceutical marketing has significantly influenced medical practice patterns. Aggressive advertising campaigns are pushing these medications.

There's a reason for this aggressive marketing.

Testosterone can't be patented. Our creator made it, which means there's no proprietary formula to protect, no exclusive rights to monetize.

Bioidentical hormones don't generate the advertising budgets that patented pharmaceuticals do.

This marketing not only shapes consumer demand but also influences medical practice patterns.

Men walk in asking for what they've seen on TV, not what their bodies actually need.

The Interconnected Nature of Sexual Health

Sexual function is a complex interplay of multiple body systems

- Cardiovascular Blood flow is essential for erectile function
- Neurological Nerve function affects sensation and response
- Hormonal Testosterone and other hormones drive desire and performance
- Psychological Mental health directly impacts sexual function
- Metabolic Energy and blood sugar control affect overall vitality

- Restoring and optimizing each of these systems naturally creates a synergistic effect that can be more powerful than any single intervention.

The Franchise Clinic Approach

Some clinics will simply give you testosterone and call it done. Write the prescription, collect the fee, and move to the next patient.

That's the franchise model.

I take a different approach because I'm focused on overall health. Diabetes harms blood vessels and nerves, both of which are crucial for achieving erections. Obesity leads to plaque buildup, reducing blood flow and erectile quality.

These conditions don't just hurt you in the bedroom. They're disease processes that need proper management.

That's why all my patients are required to have their own primary care physician. The PCP handles metabolic issues like obesity and diabetes. By the time patients see me, someone else has addressed those foundational problems.

I stay in my sandbox —hormone optimization.

NUTRITIONAL OPTIMIZATION FOR SEXUAL HEALTH

The Sexual Health Diet Foundation

Macronutrient Balance

- Protein 1.2-1.6g per kg body weight for hormone production
- Healthy Fats 25-35% of calories for hormone synthesis
- Complex Carbohydrates 45-55% for sustained energy
- Fiber 25-35g daily for cardiovascular health

Foods That Enhance Sexual Function

Nitric Oxide Boosters

Watermelon is rich in citrulline, which converts to arginine in the body. Dark, leafy greens like spinach and arugula are high in nitrates, which support blood flow. Beets are an excellent source of dietary nitrates, which support vascular health. Pomegranate contains antioxidants that support vascular health and circulation. Dark chocolate contains flavonoids that improve blood flow and endothelial function.

Testosterone-Supporting Foods

Oysters are the highest dietary source of zinc, an essential nutrient for testosterone production. Lean red meat provides zinc, vitamin B12, and creatine, which support hormone synthesis. Eggs are a complete protein source and a rich source of vitamin D, which supports testosterone production. Tuna is rich in vitamin D and protein, both of which are essential for maintaining hormone health. Brazil nuts are an excellent source of selenium, which supports thyroid and testosterone function.

Anti-Inflammatory Foods

Fatty fish, such as salmon, mackerel, and sardines, provide omega-3 fatty acids that help reduce inflammation. Berries, including blueberries and strawberries, are rich in powerful antioxidants. Nuts and seeds, such as almonds, walnuts, and flaxseed, offer healthy fats and essential nutrients. Extra virgin olive oil provides healthy monounsaturated fats with anti-inflammatory properties. Turmeric is a potent anti-inflammatory compound that supports overall health.

Foods and Habits to Avoid

Sexual Function Inhibitors

Processed foods high in trans fats and additives damage vascular health and hormone production. Excessive sugar causes inflammation and blood sugar spikes that impair sexual function. Refined carbohydrates lead to insulin resistance and metabolic dysfunction. Excessive alcohol suppresses testosterone production and sexual performance. High-sodium foods contribute to hypertension and vascular damage.

Specific Dietary Pitfalls

Soy products may interfere with testosterone, though this claim remains controversial in research. Fried foods promote inflammation and arterial damage, which can impair blood flow. Artificial sweeteners may disrupt the gut microbiome and metabolic health. Excessive caffeine intake can raise cortisol levels and disrupt hormone balance. Trans fats directly damage blood vessels and impair erectile function.

The Lifestyle Factors That Actually Matter

When a man comes to me with his metabolic issues already managed by his PCP, and we begin hormone optimization, one lifestyle factor consistently impacts results more than others.

Alcohol

Men need to limit their intake if they expect to utilize testosterone's benefits fully.

Sleep also plays a role. Proper amounts of good REM sleep improve overall health. It's not critical to testosterone therapy success specifically, but it matters for the whole person.

And that's ultimately what this is about.

Strategic Supplementation

Core Sexual Health Supplements

Generally, supplement companies operate without proper oversight. Many literally fail to provide what is on their label, and they are legally allowed to do so. In my practice, we use only products verified by a third party to contain the ingredients listed on their labels. We offer our clients physician-grade supplements that are proven to contain what they claim on their labels.

I recommend all men on Hormone Replacement Therapy to take Medical Grade Zinc Glycinate and Hormone Protect.

These supplements are designed to help with the metabolism of testosterone to estrogen. Low zinc levels cause more testosterone to be converted to estrogen. Men need some estrogen and it comes from the metabolism of testosterone, but we don't want "too" much estrogen as it can lead to "man boobs" and belly fat.

Hormone Protect can further help reduce the risk of atherosclerosis, improve prostate health, and help guard against prostate enlargement, a condition known as benign prostatic hypertrophy. Research has shown that un-metabolized estrogen accumulates in prostate tissue in men as they get older.

In the event that we are out of Hormone Protect, we recommend taking DIM. DIM is the main ingredient in Hormone Protect. This can be purchased the same way as Hormone Protect.

We carry both of these supplements in office. They can also be ordered through our website. If purchasing in office, we are able to take 10% off for all Hormone Program Patients! Alternatively, you can register online to order through the direct link below.

Dosing recommendations:

- Zinc- 1 capsule daily
- Hormone Protect- 2 capsules daily
- DIM- 2 capsules Daily

https://www.wholescripts.com/register/
Enter referral code: RESTORE.
Enter "Ibrahim" in the box requesting the Providers last name.
Enter your email address.
Follow the prompts to create your account.

Vitamin D3

Dosage	2,000-5,000 IU daily (note Vitamin D3 cannot be absorbed without also taking vitamin K2)
Benefits	Testosterone production, mood enhancement
Testing	Aim for blood levels 40-60 ng/mL
Timing	With a fat-containing meal for absorption

Zinc

Dosage	15-30mg daily
Benefits	Testosterone production, immune function
Form	Zinc picolinate for best absorption
Timing	Between meals or before bed

Magnesium

Dosage	400-600mg daily
Benefits	Testosterone support, sleep quality, stress reduction
Form	Magnesium glycinate for best tolerance
Timing	Before bed for sleep benefits

Omega-3 Fatty Acids

Dosage	2-3g combined EPA/DHA daily
Benefits	Anti-inflammatory, cardiovascular health
Source	High-quality fish oil or algae-based
Testing	Omega-3 index testing available

Advanced Supplementation

L-Arginine

The recommended dosage is 3-6 grams daily for optimal results. L-Arginine offers benefits by increasing nitric oxide production and enhancing blood flow. Take it between meals for best absorption and effectiveness. It works well in combination with L-Citrulline for enhanced vascular benefits.

Ashwagandha

The recommended dosage is 300-600 milligrams daily for therapeutic effects. Ashwagandha provides benefits through stress reduction and support for testosterone levels. Use a standardized extract, such as KSM-66, for consistent quality and potency. Take it with meals to reduce the risk of stomach upset.

D-Aspartic Acid

The recommended dosage is 3 grams daily for testosterone support. D-Aspartic Acid may boost testosterone production in some men. Cycle it with 12 weeks on, followed by 1 week off for optimal effectiveness. It works best for men with low baseline testosterone levels.

Tongkat Ali

The recommended dosage is 200-400 milligrams daily for hormonal benefits. Tongkat Ali provides testosterone support and stress reduction benefits. Quality matters—use a standardized extract for consistent potency. Strong research evidence supports its effectiveness for male sexual health.

EXERCISE PROTOCOLS FOR SEXUAL ENHANCEMENT

Cardiovascular Training for Sexual Health

The Vascular Connection

Erectile function is essentially a vascular phenomenon. The same factors that improve cardiovascular health also enhance sexual function.

Optimal Cardio Protocol	
Frequency	4-5 days per week
Duration	30-45 minutes per session
Intensity	65-85% maximum heart rate
Types	Running, cycling, swimming, rowing

High-Intensity Interval Training (HIIT)	
Benefits	Improves VO2 max, growth hormone release
Protocol	30 seconds high intensity, 90 seconds recovery
Frequency	2-3 times per week
Duration	15-20 minutes total

Specific Benefits for Sexual Health

- Improved blood flow with enhanced circulation to all organs
- Nitric oxide production for better vascular function
- Stress reduction
- Lowering of the cortisol level
- Weight management
- Reduction of cardiovascular risk factors

RESISTANCE TRAINING FOR TESTOSTERONE

The Hormone-Exercise Connection

Resistance training is one of the most effective natural ways to boost testosterone production.

Optimal Resistance Training	
Frequency	3-4 days per week
Focus	Compound movements (squats, deadlifts, rows)
Intensity	70-85% of 1-rep max
Sets/Reps	3-4 sets of 6-8 reps for strength

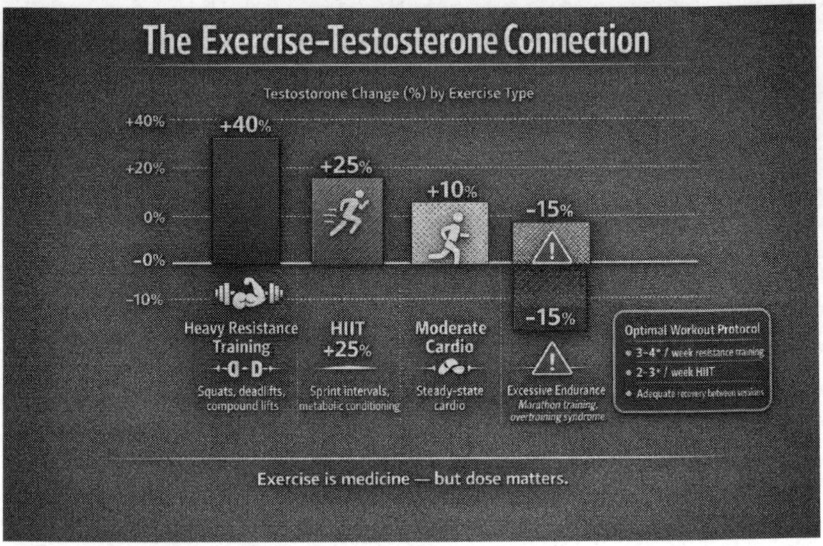

Best Exercises for Testosterone

Squats engage the largest muscle groups and trigger the release of maximum testosterone. Deadlifts are a full-body compound movement that stimulates hormone production. Pull-ups and chin-ups are compound upper-body exercises that help boost testosterone levels. Overhead press is a functional strength movement that engages multiple muscle groups. Rows develop the posterior chain and support overall strength development.

Training Variables

Rest between sets should be 2-3 minutes for heavy lifting to allow full recovery. Progressive overload refers to the gradual increase in weight or repetitions over time. Recovery requires 48-72 hours between training the same muscle groups. Sleep is crucial for recovery and hormone production after intense training.

PELVIC FLOOR TRAINING

Often overlooked but crucial for sexual function.

Understanding the Pelvic Floor	
Location	Muscles supporting pelvic organs
Function	Control urination, support erections
Problems	Weakness leads to dysfunction
Solution	Targeted strengthening exercises

Kegel Exercises for Men	
Identification	Stop urination midstream to find the muscles
Basic Exercise	Contract for 3 seconds, relax for 3 seconds
Progression	Work up to 10-second holds
Frequency	3 sets of 10, three times daily

Advanced Pelvic Floor Training
Reverse Kegels help lengthen the pelvic floor muscles and improve balance.
Breathing integration involves coordinating pelvic floor exercises with breathing patterns.
Functional movements integrate pelvic floor work with regular exercise routines.
Professional help through pelvic floor physical therapy can optimize results.

SLEEP OPTIMIZATION FOR SEXUAL HEALTH

The Sleep-Hormone Connection

Testosterone Production

Timing	80% of testosterone is produced during sleep
Deep Sleep	REM sleep is crucial for hormone release
Duration	7-9 hours, optimal for hormone production
Quality	Uninterrupted sleep is more important than duration

Sleep Architecture and Sexual Health

Stage 1-2	Light sleep, transition phases
Stage 3	Deep sleep, growth hormone release
REM Sleep	Testosterone production, psychological recovery
Cycles	4-6 complete cycles per night, optimal

Sleep Optimization Strategies

Sleep Hygiene Fundamentals

Maintain a consistent schedule with the same bedtime and wake time every day, including weekends. Create a dark environment using blackout curtains or eye masks to promote melatonin production. Maintain a cool temperature of 65-68°F, which is optimal for maintaining good sleep quality. Ensure a quiet space with white noise or earplugs if needed to minimize disruptions. Use a comfortable mattress that should be replaced every 7-10 years for proper support.

Pre-Sleep Routine

1-2 Hours Before	No screens or blue light
1 Hour Before	Relaxation activities (reading, stretching)
30 Minutes Before	Bedroom preparation, cool and dark
Bedtime	Consistent time, relaxation techniques

Sleep Disruptors to Avoid

Caffeine	No caffeine after 2 PM
Alcohol	Disrupts REM sleep, avoid 3 hours before bed
Large Meals	No heavy meals 3 hours before sleep
Exercise	No vigorous exercise 4 hours before bed
Stress	Practice stress management techniques

Advanced Sleep Strategies

Sleep Tracking

Wearable devices monitor sleep stages and quality objectively throughout the night. A sleep diary helps with tracking patterns and correlations between behaviors and sleep quality. Professional testing through a sleep study should be considered if problems persist despite interventions.

Supplements for Sleep

Melatonin	0.5-3mg, 30 minutes before bed
Magnesium	400-600mg before bed
L-Theanine	200-400mg for relaxation
Valerian Root	300-600mg natural sleep aid

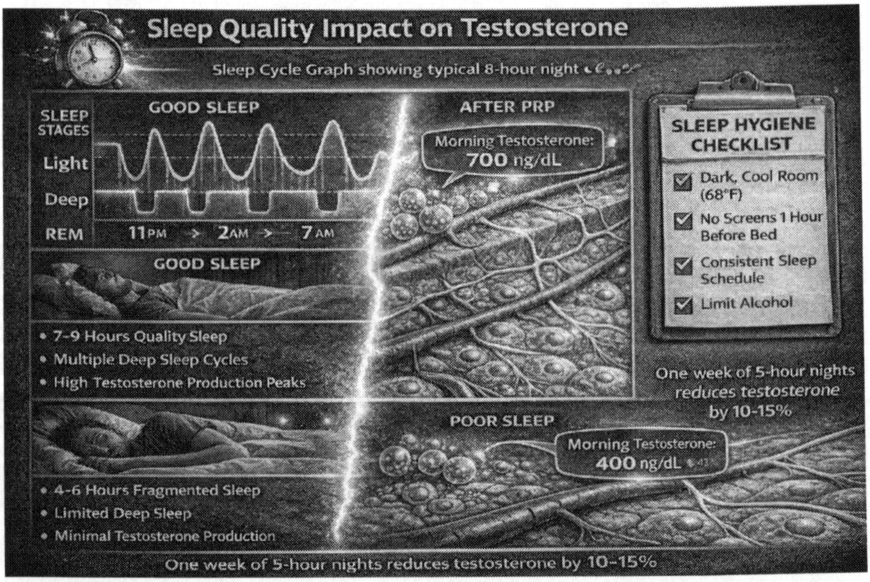

How Real Optimization Works

I'm not chasing lab numbers.

I'm listening. I want to hear the patient say they have more energy, clearer thinking, better and more satisfying erections.

How the patient feels is more important than lab values.

Here's why Testosterone levels follow a typical dosing curve. They're never truly "level." The hormone rises, then falls. Trying to maintain one specific number is impossible and misses the point entirely.

Most patients don't experience the ups and downs. When they do, I adjust the dose and schedule to minimize any peak and valley symptoms.

This is clinical medicine, not mathematics.

STRESS MANAGEMENT AND MENTAL HEALTH

The Stress-Sexual Function Connection

Physiological Impact

Cortisol elevation directly suppresses testosterone production and sexual function. Sympathetic activation reduces blood flow to sexual organs during stress responses. Inflammation creates a hostile environment for sexual function and hormone production. Sleep disruption interferes with hormone production and recovery processes.

Psychological Impact

Performance anxiety creates a self-perpetuating cycle of dysfunction and worry. Reduced libido occurs as stress decreases sexual interest and desire. Relationship strain affects intimacy and communication between partners. Self-esteem issues develop as sexual problems worsen stress levels over time.

Effective Stress Management Techniques

Mindfulness and Meditation

Daily Practice	10-20 minutes daily minimum
Types	Mindfulness, transcendental, loving-kindness
Apps	Headspace, Calm, Insight Timer
Benefits	Reduced cortisol, improved focus

Breathing Techniques

Box Breathing	4 counts in, hold, out, hold
4-7-8 Breathing	Inhale 4, hold 7, exhale 8
Coherent Breathing	5 seconds in, 5 seconds out
Practice	5-10 minutes several times daily

Physical Stress Release

Progressive muscle relaxation involves systematically tensing and releasing muscle groups throughout the body. Yoga combines movement, breathing, and mindfulness for comprehensive stress reduction. Tai chi offers gentle movement combined with meditation for mind-body balance—massage therapy, whether professional or self-massage techniques, releases physical tension.

Cognitive Strategies

Cognitive Behavioral Therapy can be pursued professionally or through self-directed programs. Journaling helps you process your thoughts and emotions constructively. Gratitude practice involves focusing on the positive aspects of your life each day. Problem-solving means addressing stressors directly rather than avoiding them.

Delivery Methods That Work

I offer two primary approaches: injections and implants.

Creams and gels are secondary methods that I will discuss, but their effectiveness does not compare to that of injections or implants. And they have the added downside of transferring to others. I don't want to be responsible for a four-year-old daughter developing pubic hair. Yes, that can happen, but not on my watch!

Injections are typically administered once or twice a week. Implants are placed every four months.

Both work equally well. Both cost the same. I follow up with patients in the same manner, regardless of the method.

So, I let the patient decide. Some men are scared of needles or don't want the inconvenience of drawing up doses and self-administering. They choose implants. Others are already comfortable with injections or prefer that level of control. They continue with that method.

Patient autonomy matters. This is their body, their treatment, their life.

OPTIMIZING ENVIRONMENTAL FACTORS

Reducing Endocrine Disruptors

Common Sources

Plastics containing BPA and phthalates in food containers leach endocrine disruptors into your food. Personal care products containing parabens and sulfates, such as shampoos and soaps, expose you to hormone-disrupting chemicals. Household cleaners create chemical residues and fumes that affect indoor air quality. Pesticides leave residues on non-organic produce that can accumulate in your body. Water supply often contains chlorine, fluoride, and pharmaceutical residues that may affect hormone balance.

Reduction Strategies

A high-quality filtration system removes contaminants from drinking water. Organic foods, especially those on the "Dirty Dozen" list, minimize exposure to pesticides. Natural products and chemical-free personal care items reduce your toxic load. Replace plastic food containers with glass storage containers to eliminate BPA exposure. Installing HEPA filters in living spaces improves indoor air quality.

Creating an Optimal Environment

Bedroom Optimization

EMF reduction involves minimizing the use of electronic devices, especially in the bedroom at night. Air quality can be improved through the use of plants, air purifiers, and proper ventilation. Lighting should maximize natural light during the day and provide complete darkness at night for the circadian rhythm. Temperature control involves maintaining a consistent temperature throughout the day to keep your environment cool and comfortable. Clutter reduction consists in maintaining a clean and organized space to promote mental clarity and focus.

ALCOHOL AND SUBSTANCE CONSIDERATIONS

Alcohol's Impact on Sexual Health

Acute Effects

Decreased sensitivity occurs with reduced sensation and sexual response after drinking. Impaired performance increases the risk of erectile dysfunction even in otherwise healthy men. Poor decision-making leads to risky sexual behaviors with potentially serious consequences. Dehydration affects overall function and can worsen sexual performance.

Chronic Effects

Testosterone suppression creates long-term hormone impact with continued alcohol use. Liver damage affects hormone metabolism and overall endocrine function. Cardiovascular impact reduces blood flow to the sexual organs over time. Sleep disruption leads to poor sleep quality and impairs hormone production.

Moderation Guidelines

Maximum	2 drinks per day for men
Alcohol-Free Days	At least 2 days per week
Quality	Choose lower-sugar options
Timing	Avoid alcohol close to intimate activities

Other Substances

Smoking and Nicotine

Smoking damages blood vessels, which impairs circulation to the penis. It suppresses testosterone production. It creates chronic inflammation throughout the body. But here's the good news stop smoking, and you'll see improvements within weeks. The body wants to heal itself. You just have to let it.

Recreational Drugs

Marijuana may reduce testosterone levels and affect motivation and sexual drive. Stimulants can cause erectile dysfunction through vasoconstriction and cardiovascular effects. Depressants impair sexual function by reducing arousal and performance. Prescription drugs, including some antidepressants and blood pressure medications, can affect sexual function as a side effect.

Beyond the Quick Fix

The pharmaceutical industry has sold us a narrative that sexual health problems have pharmaceutical solutions.

Take a pill thirty minutes before. Wait for the magic. Repeat as needed.

It's clean, simple, profitable.

It's also incomplete.

Those medications can work. They do work for many men. But they work best when built on a foundation of proper hormone levels.

Think about it logically. If low testosterone is causing poor blood flow, weak erections, low libido, and fatigue, a pill that temporarily increases blood flow addresses one symptom. It doesn't fix the underlying hormone deficiency affecting your entire system.

SOCIAL AND RELATIONSHIP FACTORS

Communication and Intimacy

Open Communication

Sexual desires should be openly discussed, including preferences and boundaries, with your partner. Performance concerns need to be shared, expressing anxieties without blame or judgment. Emotional needs require expression, particularly regarding emotional intimacy needs in the relationship. Relationship issues must be addressed directly rather than allowing them to fester.

Building Intimacy

Quality time means scheduling regular one-on-one time together without distractions. Physical affection should include non-sexual touch and closeness throughout the day. Emotional support involves being there for your partner during difficult times. Shared activities are opportunities to engage in mutual interests that strengthen your bond.

Professional Help

Couples therapy provides professional relationship counseling to improve communication and intimacy. Sex therapy offers specialized sexual health counseling for specific dysfunction issues. Individual therapy addresses personal problems that may be affecting your relationship. Support groups connect you with others who face similar challenges, providing mutual support.

The Symptom-Based Approach

When I optimize someone's testosterone, I'm not targeting a specific lab number. I'm targeting how they feel.

This represents a fundamental shift from typical medical practice, where doctors chase numbers on a chart. Hit this range, check the box, move on.

But testosterone levels fluctuate naturally. They rise and fall based on dosing schedules, individual metabolism, stress levels, sleep quality, and dozens of other factors.

Trying to keep someone at exactly 650 ng/dL or any other arbitrary number is both impossible and pointless.

What matters is whether the patient wakes up with energy. Whether their thinking is clear. Whether their erections are firm and satisfying. Whether they feel like themselves again.

Those are the metrics that matter.

CREATING YOUR PERSONAL OPTIMIZATION PLAN

Assessment and Goal Setting

Current State Evaluation

Health assessment begins with a comprehensive physical examination and thorough laboratory work. A lifestyle audit provides an honest assessment of current habits and behaviors. Stress evaluation identifies major stressors and their impact on your health. Relationship assessment evaluates support systems and the quality of intimate relationships.

SMART Goals

- **Specific:** Clear, defined objectives
- **Measurable:** Quantifiable outcomes
- **Achievable:** Realistic given the current situation
- **Relevant:** Aligned with your values and priorities
- **Time-bound:** Specific deadlines and milestones

Implementation Strategy

Phase 1: Foundation (Weeks 1-4)

Sleep optimization starts with establishing a consistent sleep schedule and good sleep hygiene. Basic nutrition involves eliminating obvious harmful foods and adding whole foods. Exercise introduction begins with just 3 days per week of moderate activity. Stress management starts with a simple daily meditation practice of 10-15 minutes.

Phase 2: Building (Weeks 5-12)

Supplement addition involves introducing core supplements, such as vitamin D, zinc, and magnesium. Exercise progression involves gradually increasing intensity and frequency as fitness improves. Advanced nutrition involves fine-tuning macronutrient ratios for optimal body composition. Relationship work focuses on enhancing communication patterns with your partner.

Phase 3: Optimization (Weeks 13-26)

Advanced techniques involve implementing sophisticated strategies, such as targeted supplementation. Fine-tuning means adjusting protocols based on results and feedback from your body. Integration focuses on making changes sustainable in the long term rather than on temporary fixes. Maintenance planning establishes ongoing protocols to ensure continued success.

Tracking and Adjustment

Objective Measures

Laboratory testing includes regular hormone and health panels to track biochemical changes. Physical metrics, including weight, body composition, and blood pressure, are monitored over time. Performance measures objectively assess exercise capacity and sleep quality. Sexual function is evaluated using standardized questionnaires for consistency.

Subjective Measures

Energy levels should be tracked daily to monitor energy and motivation throughout the day. Mood and stress require regular assessment of psychological well-being. Relationship satisfaction involves evaluating both partner and personal satisfaction levels. Overall quality of life is measured by assessing general life satisfaction across all domains.

Regular Review

Weekly	Review progress and make minor adjustments
Monthly	Assess primary metrics and trends
Quarterly	Comprehensive review and goal adjustment
Annually	Complete reassessment and planning

Working Within the System

I'm not trying to be everything to everyone.

I don't manage diabetes. I don't treat cardiovascular disease. I don't handle weight loss programs.

Other physicians excel in these areas, and I work collaboratively with them to achieve optimal results.

My focus is hormone optimization. That's my expertise, my specialty, my sandbox.

This collaborative approach serves patients better than trying to be a one-stop shop for all their needs. The PCP manages metabolic health. The cardiologist handles heart issues. I optimize hormones.

Together, we provide comprehensive care without relying on any single provider to handle everything.

The Synergistic Effect

When implemented together, these natural optimization strategies create a synergistic effect that can be more powerful than any single intervention. Men who adopt a comprehensive lifestyle approach often experience

Enhanced treatment results occur when medical treatments work more effectively on a healthy foundation. Faster recovery occurs with greater healing capacity and better adaptation to treatments. Sustained benefits develop through long-term maintenance of improvements. Overall wellness extends beyond sexual health to affect your entire life. Increased confidence comes from improved self-image and overall vitality.

COMMON CHALLENGES AND SOLUTIONS

Motivation and Consistency

Challenge	Maintaining motivation for lifestyle changes
Solutions	Start with small, manageable changes; Track progress and celebrate victories; Find accountability partners or support groups; Focus on how changes make you feel; Remember your why - the reasons for pursuing improvement.

Time Constraints

Challenge	Busy lifestyle limiting time for optimization
Solutions	Prioritize highest-impact activities; Combine activities (exercise while watching TV); Meal prep and planning strategies; Efficient workout routines (20-30 minutes); Schedule health activities like appointments

Social Pressures

Challenge	Social situations that conflict with health goals
Solutions	Prepare strategies for dining out; Communicate boundaries with friends and family; Find like-minded social groups; Focus on activities that support your goals; Practice saying no to unhealthy choices

The Reality of Aging

You can't perform at sixty the way you did at twenty-five.

That's not pessimism. That's biology.

However, you can perform significantly better than you do right now if your testosterone levels are appropriately optimized.

The goal isn't to turn back time. The goal is to provide your body with what it's missing, allowing it to function optimally for your current age.

That's realistic. That's achievable. That's what hormone optimization actually offers.

THE LONG-TERM PERSPECTIVE

Sustainable Change

Making It Last

Gradual implementation is often the most effective approach, as it avoids dramatic overnight changes that are difficult to sustain. Habit stacking means attaching new habits to existing routines to make adoption easier. Environmental design makes healthy choices easier by shaping your surroundings to promote them. Regular assessment means adjusting strategies as life changes and circumstances evolve. Flexibility is essential, allowing for imperfection and setbacks without abandoning progress.

Building Resilience

Stress inoculation gradually builds tolerance to challenges through controlled exposure. Recovery strategies involve planning for setbacks and preparing for recovery before they occur. Support systems include maintaining connections with individuals who provide guidance and support to help you achieve your goals. Continuous learning keeps you informed about new strategies and emerging research. Self-compassion involves being kind to yourself during difficult times, rather than engaging in self-criticism.

THE BILTMORE RESTORATIVE MEDICINE LIFESTYLE PROGRAM

At Biltmore Restorative Medicine & Aesthetics, we offer a comprehensive assessment as part of our sexual health optimization program.

Personalized Assessment

A comprehensive health evaluation begins with a complete medical and lifestyle assessment. A goal-setting session clarifies your objectives and priorities for a healthy journey. Obstacle identification anticipates and plans for challenges you're likely to face. Resource mapping identifies available tools and support systems you can access.

Customized Programming

Individual protocols are tailored to your specific needs and schedule for realistic implementation. Progressive implementation involves gradually introducing changes to prevent overwhelm. Regular monitoring provides ongoing assessment and adjustment based on your progress. Professional support gives you access to nutritionists, trainers, and counselors as needed.

Ongoing Support

Regular check-ins provide opportunities for progress reviews, allowing us to celebrate successes and address challenges. Educational resources offer continuous learning opportunities about health optimization. A professional network gives referrals to specialized providers when specific expertise is needed.

What This Means for You

If you're experiencing sexual health issues, start by questioning the narrative you've been sold.

Ask yourself Am I treating a symptom or addressing the root cause?

Get your testosterone levels checked. Not just total testosterone, but also free testosterone. Work with a physician who focuses on how you feel rather than just on your lab results.

Consider whether your overall health is being properly managed. Are you working with a PCP who's addressing metabolic issues? Are lifestyle factors like alcohol consumption being honestly evaluated?

And remember that you have choices in how you receive treatment. Injections and implants both work. The best method is the one you'll actually stick with.

Sexual health is part of overall health. Hormone optimization is a crucial aspect of sexual health. The pill you saw on TV might help, but it's not the whole answer.

The whole answer starts with understanding what your body actually needs.

INTEGRATING NATURAL AND MEDICAL APPROACHES

The most successful patients combine natural optimization strategies with appropriate medical treatments.

Enhanced Treatment Outcomes

A better baseline health ensures that treatments work more effectively from the outset. Faster recovery occurs with improved healing capacity and adaptation to treatments. Sustained results develop through long-term maintenance of treatment benefits. Reduced side effects are common because healthier patients tolerate treatments better and experience fewer complications.

Complementary Benefits

- Holistic wellness that extends beyond sexual health to improve your overall well-being.
- Increased energy provides overall vitality improvement throughout your daily life.
- A better mood develops through enhanced mental health and confidence.
- Improved relationships result from better communication and intimacy with your partner.

Real Patient Success Stories

"The lifestyle program at Biltmore transformed not just my sexual health, but my entire life. I lost 30 pounds, gained energy I hadn't felt in years, and my relationship with my wife is better than ever. The medical treatments were amazing, but the lifestyle changes made them even better."

—James, age 51

"I thought I just needed a quick fix, but Dr. Ibrahim showed me that real change requires a comprehensive approach. The nutrition and exercise program, combined with hormone optimization, gave me results I never thought possible at my age."

—Robert, age 47

YOUR ACTION PLAN

Getting Started

- **Complete Self-Assessment:** Honestly evaluate your current lifestyle
- **Set Realistic Goals:** Choose 2-3 areas to focus on initially
- **Create Support System:** Enlist family, friends, or professionals
- **Start Small:** Make one small change this week
- **Track Progress:** Use a journal or app to monitor changes

Building Momentum

- **Week 1-2:** Focus on sleep optimization
- **Week 3-4:** Add basic nutrition improvements
- **Week 5-6:** Incorporate regular exercise
- **Week 7-8:** Implement stress management techniques
- **Week 9-12:** Fine-tune and optimize

Long-Term Success

We conduct monthly reviews to assess your progress and adjust strategies as needed. Quarterly goal setting establishes new objectives every three months to maintain momentum. Annual assessments provide comprehensive health and lifestyle reviews to evaluate long-term progress. Continuous learning keeps you informed about new strategies and emerging research. Professional support remains available, so you can seek expert guidance whenever needed.

The foundation of sexual health is built on the daily choices you make about nutrition, exercise, sleep, stress management, and lifestyle. While medical treatments can yield remarkable results, they are most effective when combined with a commitment to overall wellness and a healthy lifestyle.

At Biltmore Restorative Medicine & Aesthetics, we understand that lasting transformation requires both advanced medical interventions and fundamental lifestyle optimization. Our comprehensive approach ensures that you not only achieve your sexual health goals but maintain them for years to come.

After thirty years of practice, that's the message I keep coming back to. Not because it's trendy or profitable, but because it's true.

You're not Viagra deficient. You never were.

Your journey to optimal sexual health begins with a single decision prioritizing your wellness. Every small change you make today builds toward the vibrant, confident, and healthy man you can become tomorrow.

References

Corona G, Rastrelli G, Morgentaler A, et al.
Meta-analysis of Results of Testosterone Therapy on Sexual Function Based on International Index of Erectile Function Scores.
Eur Urol. 2017;72(6)1000-1011.
PMID 28434676
https//pubmed.ncbi.nlm.nih.gov/28434676/

Isidori AM, Giannetta E, Gianfrilli D, et al.
Testosterone use in men with sexual dysfunction a systematic review and meta-analysis of randomized placebo-controlled trials.
Mayo Clin Proc. 2007;82(1)20-28.
PMID 17285782
https//pubmed.ncbi.nlm.nih.gov/17285782/

Snyder PJ, Bhasin S, Cunningham GR, et al.
Effect of Testosterone Replacement Therapy on Sexual Function and Hypogonadal Symptoms.
J Clin Endocrinol Metab. 2024;109(2)302-317.
PMID 37589949
https//pubmed.ncbi.nlm.nih.gov/37589949/

Luboshitzky R, Zabari Z, Shen-Orr Z, et al.
Disruption of the nocturnal testosterone rhythm by sleep fragmentation in normal men.
J Clin Endocrinol Metab. 2001;86(3)1134-1139.
PMID 11238497
https//pubmed.ncbi.nlm.nih.gov/11238497/

CHAPTER 7

Understanding Risks and Managing Expectations: What Every Man Should Know

Before we discuss risks and expectations, you need to understand how complex the testosterone production system is. This is why results vary, why lifestyle factors matter, and why patience is essential.

I Turn Away Patients Who Need Me Most

A man walks into my office and says, "I've heard amazing things about you. No one else has been able to help me, so I'm happy to be here."

My internal response? You've just met the next provider who won't be able to help you.

After 30 years of practicing men's sexual health, I've learned to recognize this patient immediately. They've been everywhere, tried everything, and blame everyone else.

And I turn them away.

Not to protect my practice, though that's a factor. I turn them away to protect them from spending money on treatments that won't satisfy them, no matter how well they work clinically.

Because here's what I've learned from thousands of patients your expectations determine your outcomes more than my skills ever will.

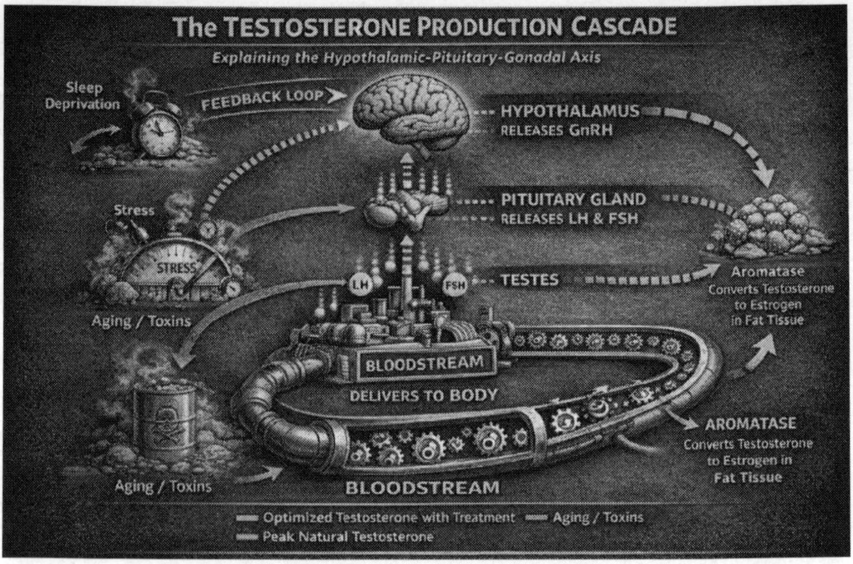

The Foundation of Informed Decision-Making

After three decades of practicing medicine and treating thousands of men, I've learned that the most satisfied patients are those who enter treatment with realistic expectations and a clear understanding of both potential benefits and risks. At Biltmore Restorative Medicine & Aesthetics, informed consent isn't just a legal requirement; it's the foundation of a successful doctor-patient relationship and optimal treatment outcomes.

This chapter will provide you with the comprehensive risk assessment and expectation management information that every man considering sexual health treatment should understand. While the treatments we offer are generally safe and effective, no medical intervention is without potential risks or limitations.

The Mind Reader Problem

The patient with unrealistic expectations thinks I'm a mind reader.

They expect me to know what they want without telling me. They expect immediate results from treatments that take months to show. They expect perfection from procedures designed to improve, not fix.

The patient with realistic expectations understands something different. They know I've treated thousands of similar cases. They know I need their feedback. They understand this is a two-way street.

After the third patient who'd "been everywhere" left a negative review despite good clinical outcomes... recognizing that while not all negative reviews stem from unrealistic expectations, this pattern taught me, I recognized the pattern. I can't meet unrealistic expectations, no matter how skilled I am.

So I stopped trying.

Improve, Never Fix

I never tell patients I'll fix their problem.

I tell them my goal is to restore function and improve the issue we're addressing.

That single word shift changes everything. It sets a realistic framework. It acknowledges limitations. It creates space for satisfaction with meaningful progress rather than disappointment at anything less than perfection.

But words alone aren't enough. Some patients hear "improve" and still think "fix" in their heads.

So I show them.

For aesthetic procedures, I manipulate their skin with my hands to demonstrate realistic outcomes. Then I exaggerate the result and explain that's what surgery might achieve, not what I can offer.

When I return to the realistic outcome, I ask whether they're okay with that result.

Then I say something out loud, "I'm now writing in your chart that I showed you both a surgical outcome and what we can realistically achieve. I'm documenting that you said our realistic outcome is acceptable. And I'm documenting that even this result isn't guaranteed."

I document this conversation in real time, while they watch me type.

Patients have not changed their answers at this moment. They already agreed. But the act of documentation changes the weight of their commitment.

They're not just nodding along anymore. They're witnessing their own agreement being recorded.

UNDERSTANDING MEDICAL RISK ASSESSMENT

The Concept of Risk-Benefit Analysis

Every medical decision involves weighing potential benefits against possible risks. This analysis must be individualized based on

Personal Risk Factors

When we assess your individual risk profile, we consider multiple interconnected factors that influence treatment safety and outcomes. Your age and overall health status form the foundation of this assessment, as they affect your body's ability to heal and respond to interventions. Existing medical conditions play a crucial role in determining which treatments are appropriate and which might pose additional risks. We carefully review your current medications and supplements because interactions can significantly impact treatment safety. Your previous surgical or treatment history provides valuable insights into how your body responds to medical interventions. Finally, lifestyle factors such as smoking, alcohol consumption, and exercise habits directly influence healing capacity and treatment success.

Treatment-Specific Factors

Treatment-specific factors that affect your risk profile include

- The invasiveness of the procedure being performed
- The complexity of the intervention and technical difficulty
- The experience level of the provider performing the treatment
- The quality and accreditation of the facility where treatment occurs
- The availability of comprehensive follow-up care and monitoring

Individual Goals and Expectations

Your individual goals and expectations are just as important as clinical factors in determining the proper treatment approach. We need to understand the outcomes you're hoping to achieve and the timeline, because this shapes which treatments make sense for your situation. Your personal tolerance for risk and uncertainty matters significantly; some men are comfortable with treatments that carry a higher risk for potentially better results, while others prefer more conservative approaches. We also carefully consider how your current problems are affecting your quality of life, as this helps us weigh whether the potential benefits of treatment justify the risks. Throughout this process, we'll discuss available alternative treatment options, ensuring you understand the full spectrum of choices before making any decisions.

RISK CATEGORIES IN SEXUAL HEALTH TREATMENT

Minimal Risk Procedures

Minimal risk procedures include:

- Routine laboratory testing and standard blood work
- Oral medications with well-established safety profiles
- Lifestyle counseling and educational interventions
- Psychological support and therapy

Low Risk Procedures

Low-risk procedures include

- Hormone replacement therapy with proper monitoring protocols
- Non-invasive treatments like Acoustic Wave Therapy
- Nutritional supplementation programs under medical guidance
- Basic sexual health screenings and evaluations

Moderate Risk Procedures

Moderate risk procedures include:

- Injection-based treatments (P-Shot®, dermal fillers)
- Minor surgical procedures
- Combination treatment protocols
- Advanced hormone optimization programs

Higher Risk Procedures

Higher risk procedures include:

- Major surgical interventions requiring significant recovery
- Experimental or unproven treatments lacking long-term data
- Procedures performed by inexperienced providers
- Treatments without proper medical supervision

Tents and Castles

Men's sexual health is tied to identity and masculinity in ways that make patience difficult.

Everything a man wants is an immediate fix. A pill that works tonight. A procedure with instant results.

So I give them a choice using a metaphor they understand.

I tell them the body isn't like a light switch. You can't turn things on and off. It's like building a brick wall. It takes time to create, and more time to make it right.

Do they want a quick fix, like a tent? Or do they want me to build a castle? Most choose the castle. Then I test their commitment.

For growth hormone enhancement, I require a six-month minimum commitment before I'll prescribe it. The treatment isn't inexpensive, but it's effective. The body takes several months to respond.

I don't want them quitting after two months, saying nothing worked when I told them it takes up to six months.

In reality, they'll see changes in three to four months. By six months, their friends will ask what they're doing because they look great.

I tell them that timeline upfront.

Why set expectations at six months when results appear earlier? Human nature. And under-promising with over-delivering.

The unrealistic patient gets upset when they don't see immediate results, even after I've explained the timeline and they've agreed to multiple treatments.

The realistic patient trusts the plan I've laid out. They understand combinations of treatments over time.

SPECIFIC RISKS BY TREATMENT TYPE

Hormone Replacement Therapy Risks

Testosterone Replacement Therapy (TRT)

Common Side Effects (5-15% of patients)

- Acne from increased oil production and breakouts
- Fluid retention with mild swelling, especially in extremities
- Sleep disturbances during the initial adjustment period
- Mood changes, including irritability or emotional fluctuations, occur during the adjustment
- Injection site reactions with redness, swelling, or discomfort

Uncommon Side Effects (1-5% of patients)

While less common than the typical side effects, some men experience additional effects that require monitoring and management. Gynecomastia, or breast tissue development, can occur but is usually preventable with proper protocols using aromatase inhibitors. Hair loss may accelerate in men who are genetically predisposed to male pattern baldness, though testosterone doesn't cause hair loss in men who weren't already going to experience it. Voice changes are pretty rare when testosterone is adequately dosed and monitored appropriately.

Polycythemia, characterized by increased red blood cell production, requires regular monitoring through blood tests and may necessitate therapeutic phlebotomy in some cases. We also monitor for prostate changes, though current research shows that testosterone replacement therapy does not exacerbate prostate cancer.

Long-term Considerations

When considering long-term testosterone therapy, several essential factors require careful discussion and planning. Fertility impact is a significant consideration because testosterone replacement can suppress your body's natural sperm production. However, this isn't inevitable; we can prevent fertility issues by using HCG concurrently with testosterone therapy to maintain testicular function and sperm production. If you stop testosterone therapy, your body's natural testosterone production will resume its pitiful production level. We also need to monitor cardiovascular health closely, tracking blood pressure and cholesterol levels throughout treatment. Metabolic effects can include changes in insulin sensitivity and lipid profiles, which is why we conduct regular comprehensive lab work to catch any concerning trends early.

Risk Mitigation Strategies

Our risk mitigation strategies for TRT include:

- Comprehensive screening with thorough evaluation before initiating therapy
- Regular monitoring with quarterly lab work and physical examinations
- Appropriate dosing starting at the lowest effective dose
- Fertility preservation using concurrent HCG when indicated
- Ongoing patient education about benefits, risks, and expectations

P-Shot® (Priapus Shot) Risks

Common Side Effects (10-20% of patients)

Common side effects after the P-Shot® include:

- Bruising that is usually mild and resolves within 7-10 days
- Swelling with temporary inflammation lasting 2-5 days
- Discomfort with mild pain or sensitivity at injection sites
- Temporary redness at injection points that fades within hours
- Minor bleeding at injection sites immediately after the procedure

Uncommon Side Effects (1-5% of patients)

While uncommon, some patients experience side effects that extend beyond the typical recovery period. Prolonged swelling lasting more than 1 week occurs in a small percentage of patients and usually resolves with conservative management. Some men notice an irregular appearance, temporary asymmetry, or small lumps under the skin, which typically resolve on their own as the PRP integrates into the tissue. Hematoma formation, a larger collection of blood under the skin, is rare but may require drainage if it becomes significant. Excessive pain beyond what we'd typically expect after this procedure warrants evaluation to rule out an underlying issue.

Rare Complications (<1% of patients)

Rare complications of the P-Shot® include:

- Infection from bacterial contamination (rare with proper sterile technique)
- Nerve damage with temporary or permanent sensation changes
- Vascular injury involving damage to blood vessels
- Allergic reactions to anesthetic agents require immediate treatment

Factors Affecting Risk

Several key factors significantly influence the risk profile of the P-Shot® procedure. Provider experience is perhaps the most crucial variable; injectors who have performed hundreds or thousands of procedures have substantially lower complication rates than those just starting out. This isn't surprising; there's no substitute for the pattern recognition and technical skill that comes from extensive hands-on experience. Sterile technique is absolutely critical, and proper preparation dramatically reduces the risk of infection to nearly zero. Your overall health status affects healing capacity; healthier patients with good nutrition, adequate sleep, and no smoking experience fewer complications across the board. Proper injection technique is crucial, encompassing correct depth, anatomical location, and the appropriate volume. Finally, how well you follow post-procedure care instructions directly impacts your outcome and risk of complications.

Priapus Toxin® Risks

Common Side Effects (15-25% of patients)

Common side effects after Priapus Toxin® include:

- Bruising that is expected and typically resolves within one week
- Swelling with mild to moderate inflammation for 3-7 days
- Temporary weakness with a brief reduction in retraction reflex (intended effect)
- Minor discomfort at injection sites for a few days
- Redness at injection points that fades quickly

Uncommon Side Effects (1-5% of patients)

Uncommon side effects of Priapus Toxin® include:

- Prolonged effects lasting longer than expected (6+ months in some cases)
- Inadequate response requiring additional treatment
- Migration of the product if injected improperly
- Asymmetry with uneven effects requiring correction

Rare Complications (<1% of patients)

Rare complications of Priapus Toxin® include:

- Systemic effects such as weakness or flu-like symptoms
- Permanent changes with lasting alterations in function or appearance
- Severe allergic reactions requiring immediate medical attention

Contraindications

Absolute contraindications for Priapus Toxin® include:

- Neuromuscular disorders (myasthenia gravis, Lambert-Eaton syndrome)
- Active infections, whether local or systemic
- Previous allergic reactions to botulinum toxin products
- Pregnancy or breastfeeding

Acoustic Wave Therapy Risks

Common Side Effects (5-10% of patients)

Common side effects during Acoustic Wave Therapy include:

- Mild discomfort during and immediately after treatment sessions
- Temporary redness with skin irritation lasting hours to days

- Sensitivity changes with brief alterations in sensation
- Petechiae (small red spots from capillary rupture) that resolve quickly

Uncommon Side Effects (1-3% of patients)

Uncommon side effects of Acoustic Wave Therapy include:

- Bruising (rare but possible with sensitive skin or certain medications
- Prolonged discomfort with pain lasting more than 24 hours
- Skin changes, including temporary pigmentation alterations
- Numbness with temporary loss of sensation in treated areas

Rare Complications (<1% of patients)

Rare complications of Acoustic Wave Therapy include:

- Skin damage, including burns or permanent skin changes
- Nerve damage with alterations in sensation or function
- Vascular injury involving damage to blood vessels

Contraindications

Contraindications for Acoustic Wave Therapy include:

- Active cancer in the treatment area
- Blood-clotting disorders with increased bleeding risk
- Pacemakers or other electronic implanted devices
- Recent surgery in the treatment area

RestoreMore (Girth Enhancement) Risks

Common Side Effects (20-30% of patients)

RestoreMore involves more significant tissue manipulation than other treatments we offer, so its side-effect profile reflects that. Swelling is substantial and typically lasts 1-2 weeks, so patients need to plan accordingly for their schedule and activities. Bruising is extensive and can persist for 7-14 days, appearing quite dramatic initially but improving steadily. Discomfort is moderate for several days post-treatment and is managed with prescribed pain medication. Temporary asymmetry is common initially as swelling settles unevenly, but this resolves as healing progresses. You'll also experience firmness during the healing phase, which gradually softens over the first few weeks.

Uncommon Side Effects (5-10% of patients)

Uncommon side effects of RestoreMore include:

- Prolonged swelling lasting more than 3 weeks requires evaluation
- Irregular texture with lumps or bumps that may require revision
- Color changes, including temporary or persistent skin discoloration
- Tenderness persists longer than expected

Rare but Serious Complications (1-3% of patients)

While rare, serious complications can occur with RestoreMore procedures and require immediate medical attention. Infections resulting from bacterial contamination must be treated promptly with appropriate antibiotics and may sometimes require removal of the filler material. Granuloma formation is an inflammatory reaction to the filler material itself, resulting in nodules that may require surgical removal or steroid injections. Vascular occlusion is the most serious complication, the blockage of blood vessels that requires immediate intervention to prevent tissue damage. Necrosis, or tissue death from compromised blood flow, is a medical emergency requiring urgent care to minimize permanent damage.

Factors Increasing Risk

Certain patient factors significantly increase the risk of complications with RestoreMore procedures, and we must address these honestly. Smoking is the single most significant risk factor; it significantly increases complication rates and impairs healing at a cellular level. If you smoke, you need to quit at least four weeks before the procedure. Diabetes creates poor healing conditions and substantially increases infection risk, so we need your blood sugar to be well-controlled before proceeding. Blood thinners increase bleeding and bruising during and after treatment, so we may need to adjust these medications with your prescribing physician. Medication- or illness-induced immunosuppression reduces your body's ability to heal and fight infections. Generally speaking, poor overall health status increases the risk of complications across the board.

The Revenue Test

Providers who promise to "fix" things instantly should raise concerns. So should providers who order tests that don't change how they'll treat you.

I use a simple principle if a lab result won't change management, it wasn't needed.

Here's a concrete example. For men, sex hormone-binding globulin (SHBG) is essential in initial lab work. This hormone helps direct treatment. But it rarely changes, and I can't easily modify it anyway.

So I test it once, act on the result, and overcome it with my treatment protocols.

I've seen other practices include SHBG in every lab draw. They're making money per test on labs that provide no additional clinical value.

That's a red flag.

It reveals a practice optimizing for revenue rather than outcomes. They're monetizing repeat testing that doesn't change what they do for you.

When a provider orders unnecessary tests, they're either incompetent or unethical. Neither option should inspire confidence.

MANAGING REALISTIC EXPECTATIONS

Understanding Normal Variation in Results

Individual Response Variability

Not every patient responds identically to treatment. Factors affecting individual response include

Biological Factors

Your biological characteristics play a fundamental role in how you respond to sexual health treatments. Age matters significantly; younger patients typically respond better to regenerative treatments because their bodies retain greater healing capacity and cellular function. Your overall health status affects every aspect of treatment response and healing; men in better physical condition generally achieve better results with fewer complications. Genetic factors that we can't control also influence treatment response, which is why identical treatments can produce somewhat different results in different patients. Baseline hormone levels are significant because men with severely low testosterone often show more dramatic improvement than those starting from near-normal levels. Finally, your vascular health, which determines the quality of blood flow throughout your body, directly affects how well erectile function treatments will work, as erections are fundamentally a vascular phenomenon.

Lifestyle Factors

Your lifestyle choices have a profound impact on treatment outcomes, often more than patients realize. Regular exercise enhances treatment outcomes through multiple mechanisms, including improved cardiovascular health, better hormone profiles, reduced inflammation, and increased overall vitality. Quality nutrition supports healing and treatment response at a cellular level; you simply can't optimize sexual health on a poor diet. Sleep quality is absolutely crucial for healing and hormone production; most testosterone is produced during deep sleep, so chronic sleep deprivation undermines everything we're trying to accomplish. Stress management affects outcomes because chronic stress elevates cortisol, which suppresses testosterone and impairs healing. Finally, substance use matters tremendously; both alcohol and tobacco negatively impact treatment results in ways that are measurable and significant.

Psychological Factors

The psychological dimension of treatment success is often underestimated but critically important. Your expectations entering treatment significantly impact your satisfaction with outcomes; realistic expectations correlate strongly with patient satisfaction, while unrealistic expectations predict dissatisfaction, regardless of clinical results. Anxiety levels matter because high anxiety can directly interfere with sexual function improvements through physiological stress responses. Relationship quality significantly influences treatment success, as partner support enhances outcomes, while relationship conflict undermines them. Your motivation and commitment to the treatment plan affect adherence to protocols and lifestyle changes that optimize results. Finally, your overall mental health status, including depression, anxiety disorders, or other psychological conditions, impacts both sexual function and treatment response.

REALISTIC OUTCOME EXPECTATIONS BY TREATMENT

Hormone Optimization Realistic Outcomes

Timeline for Improvement

Week 1-2	Initial energy improvements may begin.
Week 3-4	Mood and motivation changes become noticeable.
Week 6-8	Physical changes (muscle mass, fat loss) begin.
Months 3-6	Sexual function improvements typically peak.
Months 6-12	Full benefits realized and stabilized.

Expected Improvements

Energy levels	60-80% of patients report significant improvement.
Mood and motivation	70-85% see meaningful enhancement.
Muscle mass	5-15% increase with proper exercise.
Fat loss	10-20% reduction in body fat percentage.
Sexual function	75-90% experience meaningful improvement.

Limitations

Let me clarify what hormone optimization can and cannot do. This is not a fountain of youth, and it cannot reverse all the effects of aging; anyone who promises otherwise is deceiving you. Hormone optimization requires ongoing maintenance; it's not a one-time fix but a long-term commitment to sustained treatment for continued benefits. Individual variation in response is significant; some men respond dramatically while others see more modest improvements, and we can't always predict who will fall into which category. Side effects are possible with any medical treatment and require careful monitoring and management throughout therapy.

P-Shot® Realistic Outcomes

Functional Improvements

- **Erectile quality:** 70-80% of patients report firmer erections.
- **Sensitivity enhancement:** 80-90% experience increased sensation.
- **Performance duration:** Modest improvements in stamina.
- **Natural response:** Enhanced spontaneous erectile function.

Size Enhancement Expectations

Realistic Limitations

I need you to understand the realistic limitations of P-Shot® therapy before you commit to it. The improvements you'll see are meaningful and valuable, but they're not dramatic. This isn't going to transform you into a different person sexually. This is a gradual process where results develop over months, not days or weeks, requiring patience and realistic expectations. Individual variation in response is substantial; some men experience significant improvement while others see more modest changes, and we can't predict with certainty where you'll fall on that spectrum. Maintenance is necessary because the benefits gradually diminish over time without periodic retreatment, typically every 12 to 18 months.

Acoustic Wave Therapy Realistic Outcomes

Functional Improvements

Functional improvements from Acoustic Wave Therapy include:

- **Erectile function:** 60-75% of patients see significant improvement in firmness
- **Natural response:** Reduced dependence on ED medications over time
- **Duration Improved:** ability to maintain erections throughout sexual activity
- **Sensitivity:** Enhanced sensation through improved nerve function and blood flow

Timeline and Duration

Initial response	Some improvement within 2-4 weeks.
Peak benefits	Maximum improvement at 3-6 months.
Duration	Benefits typically last 1-2 years.
Maintenance	An annual series is recommended for sustained benefits.

Best Candidates

Acoustic Wave Therapy is most effective for specific patient profiles. Men with vascular erectile dysfunction, meaning circulation-related problems, respond most effectively because the treatment directly addresses the root cause by improving blood vessel function. Mild to moderate cases show better results than severe dysfunction; if the problem is too advanced, acoustic waves alone may not be sufficient. Younger men generally experience better outcomes because their bodies retain greater regenerative capacity and vascular health. Overall, good health predicts better response to treatment across the board.

RestoreMore Realistic Outcomes

Enhancement Results

Enhancement results with RestoreMore include:

- **Girth increase:** 40-60% improvement in circumference for most patients
- **Immediate visibility:** Results are apparent immediately after treatment
- **Natural appearance:** Maintained with proper technique and realistic volume
- **Partner satisfaction:** Typically increases with noticeable enhancement

Timeline

Immediate Results are visible right after the procedure.

1-2 Weeks	Swelling subsides, results more apparent.
1-3 Months	Final settling and optimization.
Duration	12-24 months, typical longevity.

Important Limitations

RestoreMore has significant limitations you need to understand before proceeding. This is a temporary solution, not a permanent enhancement; the filler material gradually breaks down over time. Maintenance is necessary, with touch-up treatments needed every 9-18 months to maintain results. Individual variation significantly affects longevity; some patients experience 18-24 months of longevity from a single treatment, while others require touch-ups sooner. Migration of the product is possible if it moves from the original injection sites, though this is minimized with proper technique.

Vetting Your Provider

Online reviews can be manufactured. Websites can look impressive. Marketing can sound authoritative.

So how do you actually vet a sexual health provider?

Start with online reviews and years in business. Providers can't enter these themselves. Look for patterns over time, not just star ratings.

Ask where they were educated. Not just medical school, but specific training in the treatments they offer.

Ask if they're practicing within their formal training. I'm a urologist who trained specifically in male genital and urinary systems. That's direct alignment.

If your provider is a chiropractor offering hormone therapy, that's a different story. Not necessarily wrong, but worth understanding the gap between their training and their practice.

Look for experience and reputation, but verify both.

New providers can be honest and capable. But years of experience with thousands of patients create pattern recognition you can't get from textbooks.

FACTORS THAT INFLUENCE TREATMENT SUCCESS

Pre-Treatment Optimization

Health Status Optimization

Pre-treatment health optimization includes:

- **Cardiovascular health:** Blood pressure and cholesterol management
- **Blood sugar control:** Optimal glucose levels for healing
- **Weight management:** Achieving a healthy BMI
- **Smoking cessation:** Quitting at least 4 weeks before procedures

Lifestyle Preparation

Proper lifestyle preparation before treatment significantly improves outcomes and reduces the risk of complications. Establish a regular exercise program before beginning treatment; even moderate activity, such as walking 30 minutes daily, can make a measurable difference in your healing capacity. Optimize your nutrition by adopting healthy eating patterns that prioritize whole foods, sufficient protein, and a variety of vegetables. Ensure proper sleep habits. Implement stress-reduction techniques, such as meditation, deep breathing, or other methods that work for you, to manage daily stress effectively. Finally, eliminate alcohol and recreational drugs for at least two weeks before any procedure to optimize healing.

Psychological Preparation

Psychological preparation is just as necessary as physical preparation. Develop realistic expectations by truly understanding what outcomes are achievable versus what's wishful thinking. This conversation needs to happen before treatment, not after. Ensure you have an adequate support system for emotional support during the process; this journey is easier with people who understand what you're going through. Work on communication with your partner if you're in a relationship, because enhanced intimacy requires openness and vulnerability. Address any significant mental health issues like anxiety or depression before treatment, as these can interfere with outcomes. Finally, assess your motivation honestly. Are you genuinely committed to the lifestyle changes and follow-through necessary for optimal results?

During Treatment Factors

Provider Expertise

When selecting a provider for sexual health treatment, several factors should guide your decision. Experience level matters tremendously; find out how many procedures the provider has performed and how many years they've been practicing in this specific field. The training background encompasses specialized education and certification, not just general medical training, but also particular expertise in the treatments you're considering. Facility quality encompasses safety standards, sterility protocols, accreditation, and the overall professionalism of the environment. Patient outcomes should be documented through success rates and complication data; any provider unwilling to discuss their outcomes should raise red flags. Finally, assess communication style and rapport; you need a provider who addresses your concerns effectively and makes you feel comfortable asking questions.

Patient Compliance

Treatment compliance requires:

- Following all pre- and post-procedure guidelines carefully
- Taking prescribed medications exactly as directed
- Respecting activity restrictions during the healing period
- Attending all scheduled follow-up appointments
- Communicating honestly with your provider about any concerns

Post-Treatment Factors

Recovery Optimization

During the recovery period:

- **Rest and recovery:** Allow adequate healing time after procedures
- **Activity modification:** Gradually return to normal activities as tolerated
- **Wound care:** Properly care for injection sites or incisions
- **Pain management:** Use prescribed medications as directed for comfort
- **Monitor for complications:** Watch for any signs of problems and report them

Long-term Maintenance

Long-term maintenance includes:

- **Lifestyle continuation:** Maintain healthy habits established during treatment
- **Regular monitoring:** Keep all follow-up appointments as scheduled
- **Touch-up treatments:** Pursue maintenance procedures when needed
- **Ongoing optimization:** Continue attention to health and wellness

The Vulnerability Requirement

The first thing you should do before calling any clinic is get ready to be vulnerable.

Not vulnerable to sharing your problem. That's expected.

Vulnerable to hearing what the provider offers, even if it's not what you want to hear.

I tell new patients my job is to build their trust. To do that, I need them to give me some initial trust. Let me do what I know has worked for others, tweaked to their specific situation. This is the partnership model.

You bring vulnerability and willingness to follow guidance. I bring experience and customized protocols. Together, we work toward realistic outcomes over appropriate timelines.

The patient who walks in having already decided what they want rarely succeeds. They're not looking for a partner. They're looking for someone to execute their predetermined plan.

The patient who walks in ready to learn usually does well. They understand I've seen their situation hundreds of times. They're willing to trust the process while staying engaged.

Red Flags and Warning Signs – When to Seek Immediate Medical Attention

Emergency Situations

Seek immediate emergency medical attention for specific symptoms; call 911 or go to the nearest emergency room. A severe allergic reaction with difficulty breathing, widespread rash, or significant swelling requires immediate emergency care without delay. Signs of a serious infection, including fever over 101°F, severe pain, drainage of pus, or red streaking spreading from the treatment site, warrant urgent medical evaluation. Any chest pain or significant shortness of breath following treatment must be evaluated immediately to rule out serious complications. Severe bleeding that doesn't stop with direct pressure requires emergency intervention. Loss of consciousness, altered mental status, or neurological symptoms like numbness or weakness demand immediate emergency response.

Urgent (Same Day) Situations

Contact your provider the same day for:

- Severe pain not controlled by prescribed medications
- Excessive swelling that worsens after 48 hours
- Unusual discharge, including pus or abnormal drainage
- Spreading redness beyond the treatment area
- Fever over 101.5°F, suggesting possible infection

Prompt (Within 24-48 Hours) Situations

Schedule a follow-up appointment for:

- Increasing pain that gets worse instead of better
- Persistent swelling that doesn't improve after one week
- Low-grade fever below 101.5°F lasting more than 48 hours
- Unexpected side effects or concerns about your recovery
- Questions about recovery progress or timeline

Risk Mitigation Strategies

Provider Selection

Perform due diligence by:

- Verifying credentials and specialized training
- Checking experience with the specific procedure and years of practice
- Visiting the facility to assess cleanliness and professionalism
- Reviewing testimonials and patient reviews from multiple sources
- Assessing how thoroughly the provider addresses your concerns

Informed Consent Process

The informed consent process is a legal and ethical requirement that protects both you and your provider. A comprehensive discussion must thoroughly cover all risks, benefits, and alternative treatment options, rather than merely checking boxes on a form. Written documentation includes detailed consent forms that you should actually read, not just sign, before agreeing to treatment. You need adequate opportunity to ask questions and receive clear, honest answers to all your concerns without feeling rushed. Take the time you need to consider the decision; no reputable provider should pressure you to make a decision immediately. Finally, we verify your understanding by asking you to explain what you understand about the treatment, risks, and expected outcomes.

Preparation Optimization

Pre-treatment assessment includes:

- Complete medical evaluation and health screening
- Comprehensive medication and supplement review
- Lifestyle optimization addressing modifiable risk factors
- Baseline laboratory testing for monitoring purposes
- Physical examination documenting baseline status

What Success Actually Looks Like

Success in sexual health treatment isn't about perfect outcomes.

It's about meaningful improvement that aligns with realistic expectations.

The most satisfied patients aren't necessarily those with the best clinical results. They're the ones who understood the possibilities and limitations before starting.

They trusted the timeline I established. They followed through on multiple treatments when needed. They gave feedback so I could adjust protocols.

They built the castle instead of demanding a tent that looked like one.

Sexual health treatment is a partnership. Your participation influences outcomes as much as my expertise.

The patient who expects me to read their mind and deliver perfection immediately will be disappointed, regardless of what I do.

The patient who comes ready to be vulnerable, trust the process, and commit to realistic timelines usually leaves satisfied.

Not because I'm exceptional, though I am experienced.

Because they understood from the beginning what we were building together.

LEGAL AND ETHICAL CONSIDERATIONS

Informed Consent Requirements

Legal Standards

Valid informed consent requires:

- **Disclosure:** All material risks must be disclosed to the patient
- **Understanding:** Patient must demonstrate comprehension
- **Voluntariness:** Decision made without coercion or pressure
- **Competence:** Patient has the capacity to make medical decisions
- **Documentation:** Written record of the consent process

Ethical Principles

Key ethical principles include:

- **Autonomy:** Respecting patients' right to make their own decisions
- **Beneficence:** Acting in patients' best interest at all times
- **Non-maleficence:** Following the "no harm" principle
- **Justice:** Ensuring fair and equitable treatment access

Patient Rights and Responsibilities

Patient Rights

Your patient rights include:

- **Information:** Right to complete and accurate information about treatments
- **Choice:** Right to accept or refuse treatment without penalty
- **Privacy:** Confidential handling of all medical information
- **Respect:** Dignified and courteous treatment at all times

Patient Responsibilities

Your patient responsibilities include:

- **Honest communication:** Provide accurate and complete medical history
- **Compliance:** Follow treatment protocols and instructions as prescribed
- **Payment:** Meet financial obligations as agreed upon
- **Respect:** Treat medical staff and other patients courteously
- **Communication:** Report any problems or concerns promptly

INSURANCE AND FINANCIAL CONSIDERATIONS

Insurance Coverage Limitations

Typically Not Covered

Services typically NOT covered by insurance:

- Cosmetic enhancement procedures
- Elective sexual health treatments
- Experimental or investigational treatments
- Treatments for sexual satisfaction rather than dysfunction

Potentially Covered

Services potentially covered by insurance

- Treatment of diagnosed medical conditions
- Hormone replacement for documented deficiency
- Treatments for erectile dysfunction
- Psychological counseling for sexual problems

Documentation Requirements

Insurance documentation requires:

- Medical necessity documentation establishing the need for treatment
- Documentation of failed conservative treatment attempts
- Objective evidence of dysfunction supporting the claim
- Clear provider recommendations and treatment rationale

Financial Planning

Cost Considerations

Treatment costs include:

- Initial evaluation Consultation and testing costs
- Treatment costs Procedure and medication expenses
- Follow-up care Monitoring visits and lab work
- Maintenance treatments Costs for sustaining results over time

Payment Options

Payment options available:

- Cash payment (may be discounted for payment in full)
- Financing plans through medical financing companies
- In-house payment arrangements
- Health savings accounts (HSA/FSA)
- Credit cards for convenient payment processing

THE BILTMORE RESTORATIVE MEDICINE APPROACH TO RISK MANAGEMENT

Comprehensive Risk Assessment

Pre-Treatment Evaluation

The initial evaluation is comprehensive and designed to gather all necessary information for safe and effective treatment planning. We begin with a detailed medical history that covers not just your sexual health concerns but your complete health background, including past surgeries, medical conditions, medications, and family history. A thorough physical examination evaluates the relevant systems and provides baseline measurements for each system. Laboratory testing includes comprehensive blood work and any additional diagnostic tests necessary to assess your current health status and identify potential issues that may impact treatment safety. We perform individualized risk assessment based on all the information gathered. Finally, we develop a customized treatment plan based on your specific needs, goals, and risk profile.

Informed Consent Process

Treatment planning involves more than just deciding which procedure to perform. We have a detailed discussion that comprehensively reviews all risks and benefits, without glossing over any details or minimizing potential downsides. You will receive written materials, including educational resources and detailed consent forms, all of which are explained in plain language. Take these home and read them carefully. We provide adequate time for questions and answers, addressing all your concerns thoroughly without rushing through the conversation. We present alternative options and compare them with our recommended approach, so you understand why we're recommending it. Ultimately, we establish a realistic timeline for treatment progression and expected outcomes tailored to your specific situation.

SAFETY PROTOCOLS

During Treatment

During treatment implementation:

- **Sterile technique:** Hospital-grade infection control procedures
- **Emergency preparedness:** Immediate access to emergency care if needed
- **Monitoring:** Continuous observation during and after procedures
- **Comfort measures:** Pain control and anxiety management
- **Documentation:** Detailed records of all aspects of treatment

Post-Treatment Care

Post-treatment care includes:

- **Recovery:** monitoring Immediate post-procedure observation
- **Detailed instructions:** Written post-care guidelines to follow at home
- **Emergency contact:** 24/7 access for urgent concerns
- **Follow-up scheduling:** Appropriate monitoring appointments
- **Complication management:** Clear protocols for addressing problems

QUALITY ASSURANCE

Outcome Tracking

Quality assurance is built into every aspect of our practice. We regularly assess patient satisfaction through surveys and direct feedback, using this information to continually improve our protocols and communication. Complication rates are systematically tracked and analyzed to identify any patterns or areas for improvement. Effectiveness is measured using standardized outcome measures that enable us to evaluate whether treatments are achieving their intended results objectively. We implement continuous improvement by regularly reviewing outcome data and making protocol adjustments based on the insights gained. Provider training is ongoing, ensuring that our entire team maintains current knowledge and skills through continuing education.

Making Informed Decisions

Questions to Ask Your Provider

About Risks

What are the most common complications for this procedure? What is your personal complication rate? How do you handle complications when they occur? What emergency protocols do you have in place? How many of these procedures have you personally performed?

About Benefits

What realistic outcomes can I expect? How long will results typically last? What percentage of patients are satisfied with the results? What if I'm not happy with the outcome? Are there alternative treatments to consider?

About the Process

What does the procedure involve exactly? How long is the recovery period? What restrictions will I have during recovery? When can I expect to see results? What follow-up care is included?

RED FLAGS IN PROVIDER SELECTION

Warning Signs to Avoid

Certain warning signs should make you walk away from a provider immediately. Unrealistic promises that guarantee specific outcomes are a huge red flag; no honest provider can guarantee results in medicine. High-pressure sales tactics suggest that the provider prioritizes closing the sale over your well-being. Inadequate consultation, where the evaluation feels rushed, indicates the provider isn't taking the time to assess your situation correctly. Incomplete informed consent, with insufficient risk disclosure, is not only unethical but also potentially illegal. Finally, lack of proper credentials or qualifications is an absolute deal-breaker; verify everything before proceeding.

The Choice You're Really Making

When you choose a sexual health provider, you're not just choosing their skills.

You're choosing whether to be the kind of patient who succeeds.

You can walk in expecting miracles, demanding instant results, and blaming providers when reality doesn't live up to your imagination.

Or you can walk in ready to hear hard truths, commit to appropriate timelines, and participate actively in your own care.

I'll turn away the first patient every time. Not because I don't want to help them, but because I'm unable to. Their expectations make success impossible.

The second patient? That's who I built my practice for. That's the partnership that changes lives.

DECISION-MAKING FRAMEWORK

Step 1: Self-Assessment

Begin with a personal assessment:

- Clearly define your goals and expectations for treatment
- Assess your risk tolerance and what complications you're willing to accept
- Evaluate your financial capacity for the required investment
- Consider timing and life circumstances for treatment feasibility

Step 2: Provider Research

Provider research should include:

- Thoroughly researching potential providers before making decisions
- Scheduling consultations with multiple providers to compare
- Comparing approaches and recommendations from different practitioners
- Verifying credentials and experience through independent sources

Step 3: Information Gathering

Information gathering includes:

- Asking detailed questions about risks and benefits
- Requesting written materials for review at your own pace
- Seeking second opinions when appropriate for major decisions
- Researching treatment options independently

Step 4: Decision Making

Decision-making process:

- Take adequate time to consider all information
- Discuss with trusted friends or family for perspective
- Consider long-term implications of treatment decisions
- Make decisions without external pressure or rushed timelines

Step 5: Preparation and Planning

Treatment preparation involves:

- Optimizing health status before treatment begins
- Arranging for support during recovery from family or friends
- Planning for time away from work and activities
- Preparing financially for all treatment-related costs

CONCLUSION: INFORMED CHOICES LEAD TO BETTER OUTCOMES

Understanding risks and maintaining realistic expectations are fundamental to achieving satisfaction with sexual health treatments. While the treatments we offer at Biltmore Restorative Medicine & Aesthetics are generally safe and effective, they are medical procedures with inherent risks and limitations.

After 30 years and thousands of patients, I've learned that the treatment you choose matters less than the expectations you bring and the partnership you're willing to build.

Everything else is just details.

The key to success lies in

- **Thorough Education:** Understanding all aspects of treatment
- **Realistic Expectations:** Accepting achievable outcomes
- **Proper Preparation:** Optimizing health and circumstances
- **Provider Selection:** Choosing experienced, qualified professionals
- **Commitment to Care:** Following through with treatment protocols and follow-up

Remember that sexual health treatment is a partnership between you and your medical team. Your active participation in the decision-making process, preparation, treatment, and recovery phases significantly influences your outcome and satisfaction.

At Biltmore Restorative Medicine & Aesthetics, we're committed to providing you with the information, support, and expert care needed to make informed decisions about your sexual health. Our goal is not only successful treatment but also confident and satisfied patients who achieve their personal goals safely and effectively.

The decision to pursue sexual health treatment is significant and personal. Take the time to fully understand your options, risks, and expectations. When you're ready to proceed, we're here to support you every step of the way, building castles, not tents.

References

Rasmussen JN, Haugaard SB, Rasmussen DB, et al.
Erectile Dysfunction and Risk of Cardiovascular Disease and Mortality.
Am Heart J. 2021;23550-61.PMID 33278354
https//pubmed.ncbi.nlm.nih.gov/33278354/

Masterson TA, Molina M, Ledesma B, et al.
Platelet-rich plasma for the treatment of erectile dysfunction a prospective, randomized, double-blind, placebo-controlled clinical trial.
J Urol. 2023;210(1)154-161.PMID 37120727
https//pubmed.ncbi.nlm.nih.gov/37120727/

Porst H, Burnett A, Brock G, et al.
SOP conservative (medical and mechanical) treatment of erectile dysfunction.
J Sex Med. 2013;10(1)130-171. PMID 23343165
https//pubmed.ncbi.nlm.nih.gov/23343165/

CHAPTER 8

Investment in Yourself: The Real Cost of Sexual Health Treatment

The Hidden Economics of Sexual Health Optimization

I watch patients pull up in six-figure automobiles. They're wearing jewelry that costs $15,000. They take vacations that run $20,000 or more.

Then they sit in my office and tell me they can't afford sexual health treatment.

I don't know how to place a value on sexual health. I consider it priceless. A healthy sex life is secondary only to a healthy life, and you cannot have a completely healthy life without a healthy sex life.

But here's what I've learned after more than a decade in restorative medicine: when someone says they can't afford treatment, they're not doing the real math.

Understanding the True Value of Sexual Health Investment

After three decades of helping men restore their vitality and confidence, I've learned that the cost of sexual health treatment goes far beyond the financial investment. At Biltmore Restorative Medicine & Aesthetics, we regularly see men who initially hesitate about the financial commitment, only to later describe their treatment as "the best investment I've ever made." This chapter will help you understand not just the monetary costs but the comprehensive value proposition of sexual health optimization.

The Luxury Paradox

The disconnect is striking. People readily invest in luxury items but hesitate about sexual health. They'll write a check for a car upgrade without a second thought. They'll book an expensive trip on impulse.

But a $20,000 investment in restoring and optimizing comprehensive sexual health? That requires convincing.

I'm not ashamed of the investment required to deliver the services we provide. High-quality care delivered by highly trained, experienced providers costs what it costs. The figures are well justified.

What bothers me is watching what happens to the patients who drive away without investing.

THE COMPLETE COST ANALYSIS FRAMEWORK

Direct Financial Costs

Initial Investment Components

- Comprehensive evaluation including medical history, physical exam, and laboratory testing.
- Treatment procedures covering the actual medical interventions.
- Follow-up care involves ongoing monitoring, adjustments, and support.
- Maintenance treatments with periodic touch-ups or continuing care.
- Adjunct services like counseling, nutrition coaching, and fitness support.

Ongoing Financial Considerations

The ongoing financial picture includes replacement and maintenance costs for repeat treatments that help you maintain the benefits you've achieved. You'll want to factor in health optimization expenses such as supplements and lifestyle programs that support your results. There's also the opportunity for further improvement through additional treatments. Keep in mind that insurance limitations mean most of these treatments won't be covered by your health plan. Finally, consider the time investment; the value of the time you'll spend in treatment and recovery is part of the equation as well.

Hidden and Indirect Costs

Opportunity Costs

When calculating opportunity costs, consider the time away from work you'll need for appointments, procedures, and recovery. There's also the relationship investment, the time and energy you're currently spending trying to address sexual issues. Don't forget the money wasted on ineffective alternative treatments. Delayed decisions carry their own cost as problems worsen and compound over time. And perhaps most significantly, there's the quality-of-life impact; the ongoing suffering from untreated sexual health issues affects every aspect of your daily life.

Current Problem Costs

Many men don't realize the ongoing cost of NOT addressing sexual health issues:

- Relationship strain requiring counseling, therapy, or potentially leading to separation/divorce can incur high costs.
- Mental health impact, including depression and anxiety treatment costs.
- Performance medications with ongoing costs of ED drugs.

- Self-medication expenses on supplements, devices, or other attempted solutions
- Professional impact from reduced confidence and energy affecting career

The Real Costs Start Immediately

The moment someone leaves my office without receiving treatment, costs begin to accumulate.

Self-doubt becomes the first expense.

Will I be able to perform? Will I ever lust after my spouse again? Will my partner cheat on me?

These questions don't appear on any ledger. But they compound daily.

Patients talk about how sexual dysfunction affects their marriage. Women who haven't had sex or initiated intimacy in years carry that weight everywhere. The bedroom becomes a source of anxiety rather than a connection.

That anxiety doesn't stay contained.

TREATMENT-SPECIFIC INVESTMENT ANALYSIS

Hormone Optimization Investment

Initial Setup Costs

Comprehensive Evaluation $500-800

- Detailed consultation with a hormone specialist
- Complete laboratory panel (20+ markers)
- Physical examination and health assessment
- Treatment planning and goal setting

- Initial Treatment Phase $300-600 monthly
- Bioidentical hormone replacement
- Monitoring and adjustments
- Supportive medications if needed
- Regular follow-up consultations

Ongoing Investment

- Maintenance Phase $200-400 monthly
- Continued hormone replacement
- Quarterly monitoring and lab work
- Annual comprehensive evaluation
- Dosage adjustments as needed

Long-term Value Analysis

Duration: Typically lifelong once started

Total Annual Investment $2,400-4,800

Cost Per Day $6.50-13.00 daily

Comparison: Less than many men spend on coffee or supplements

Return on Investment

The returns on this investment extend across multiple dimensions of your life. Energy improvements translate directly into increased productivity and deeper engagement with work and family. The health benefits are substantial; you'll see reduced risk of cardiovascular disease, diabetes, and osteoporosis. Your overall quality of life improves as you experience enhanced mood, stronger motivation, and greater life satisfaction. Relationship benefits manifest through improved intimacy and better communication with your partner. And don't overlook the potential medical cost savings from future reductions in healthcare expenses.

P-Shot® (Priapus Shot) Investment

Procedure Cost Breakdown

Single Treatment $1,500-2,000

- Comprehensive consultation and planning
- Blood draw and PRP preparation
- Anesthesia and injection procedure
- Immediate post-procedure care
- Follow-up appointments

Value Components

- Immediate benefits with results beginning within 2-4 weeks
- Duration where benefits typically last 12-18 months
- Cost per month of $85-165 (amortized over benefit period)
- Maintenance through annual treatments for sustained benefits

Comparative Analysis

- vs. ED Medications Many men spend $200-400 monthly on ED drugs
- vs. Supplements Unproven supplements often cost $100+ monthly
- vs. Devices Vacuum pumps, rings, and devices cost hundreds, with questionable results
- vs. Surgery Surgical options cost $15,000-25,000 with higher risks

Enhancement Benefits

- Functional improvement, including better erections and sensitivity
- Natural results using the body's own healing factors

- Safety profile with minimal risk under experienced provider guidance
- Confidence boost provides psychological benefits beyond physical improvement

Priapus Toxin® Investment

Treatment Investment

- Single Session $1,200-1,800
- Consultation and treatment planning
- Anesthesia and injection procedure
- Post-treatment monitoring
- Follow-up care and assessment

Value Proposition

Immediate results with improvement visible within days, duration of 6-12 months of benefits, monthly cost of $100-300 (amortized), and unique benefits as the only treatment addressing penile shrinkage.

Confidence Investment

The psychological impact creates dramatic improvements in confidence that extend well beyond the bedroom. You'll experience enhanced intimacy and greater self-assurance in your relationship. Social confidence improves as you feel more comfortable in various situations. Additionally, the performance enhancement aspect is significant, as better erectile function and improved control contribute to an overall sense of capability and confidence.

Acoustic Wave Therapy Investment

Complete Series Cost

- Initial Series: $3,000-5,000
- 6-12 treatment sessions

- Comprehensive evaluation and planning
- Advanced acoustic wave technology
- Progress monitoring throughout

Value Analysis

Drug-free solution eliminating need for ED medications, long-lasting results with benefits typically lasting 1-2 years, annual cost of $1,500-2,500 (amortized over benefit period), and maintenance through annual series for sustained benefits.

Comparative Savings

- vs. ED Medications $2,400-4,800 annually for prescription drugs
- vs. Injection Therapy $3,000-6,000 annually for injection treatments
- vs. Surgery Penile implants cost $20,000-30,000
- Natural Approach Restores the body's natural function

RESTOREMORE™ (GIRTH ENHANCEMENT) INVESTMENT

Procedure Investment

- Treatment Cost $4,000-8,000
- Varies based on enhancement goals
- Includes consultation, procedure, and follow-up
- Premium filler materials
- Experienced injector expertise

Value Considerations

Instant results with enhancements visible immediately, lasting 12-24 months, with typical longevity. Revision options are available, including touch-ups for optimization, and the procedure is reversible, allowing for adjustments or dissolution if desired.

Confidence Value: Improved self-image and relationship satisfaction

Comparison Analysis

- vs. Surgical Enhancement $15,000-25,000 with higher risks
- vs. Ongoing Dissatisfaction Quality of life impact of body image concerns

COMPREHENSIVE TREATMENT PACKAGE INVESTMENT

The Complete Optimization Program

For optimal results, many patients opt for comprehensive treatment that combines multiple approaches.

Package Components

- Hormone Optimization $3,000-6,000 annually
- P-Shot® Series $3,000-4,000 (2 treatments yearly)
- Acoustic Wave Therapy $3,000-5,000 annually
- Priapus Toxin® $2,400-3,600 (2-3 treatments yearly)
- RestoreMore™ $4,000-8,000 (as desired)
- Total Annual Investment $15,000-25,000

Package Discounts

Combination savings offering 10-20% discount for multiple treatments, loyalty programs with reduced costs for ongoing patients, and payment plans providing financing options to spread costs.

Return on Investment Analysis

Quantifiable Benefits

- Relationship savings avoid counseling, therapy, and separation costs
- Career enhancement through increased confidence, leading to professional advancement
- Health improvements reducing the risk of chronic diseases
- Medication savings, eliminating ED drugs and related costs

Quality of Life Benefits

The quality-of-life benefits are perhaps the most profound, though they're harder to quantify. Confidence enhancement improves your self-esteem and makes social interactions more enjoyable and natural. Relationship improvement manifests through better intimacy and more open communication with your partner. You'll experience renewed energy and vitality, enhancing your overall engagement with life. Mental health improvements reduce anxiety and depression. Physical health benefits contribute to improved overall wellness and disease prevention.

THE COMPOUND INTEREST PROBLEM IN REVERSE

Now consider the opposite scenario.

A 52-year-old man is experiencing these issues. His testosterone is declining, his libido has vanished, and he's struggling with erectile dysfunction. He decides to wait three years before starting treatment.

What's compounding during those three years?

He's depriving his marriage of a healthy sex life. His partner isn't happy. Waiting will not make things better.

The decline accelerates with age. The older someone is when the five-year clock starts, the more rapid the deterioration.

He gains fat, particularly around the midsection. His muscle mass deteriorates. He alienates his spouse more. Pre-diabetes rates go up. Cardiovascular disease risk soars. Bone density decreases.

These aren't just quality-of-life issues. These are significant medical expenses that are likely to occur.

Who wouldn't pay $20,000 to avoid a heart attack or the metabolic complications of untreated hormonal decline?

The Insurance Illusion

Here's the psychological barrier that trips up most people.

Insurance has conditioned people to think healthcare should cost no more than $20 out of pocket per visit.

They fail to grasp that when insurance is paying, the actual cost of care is significantly more than their $20 copay. They've lost touch with what quality healthcare actually costs.

But they accept paying $800 for new tires without question. They know car insurance won't cover that expense.

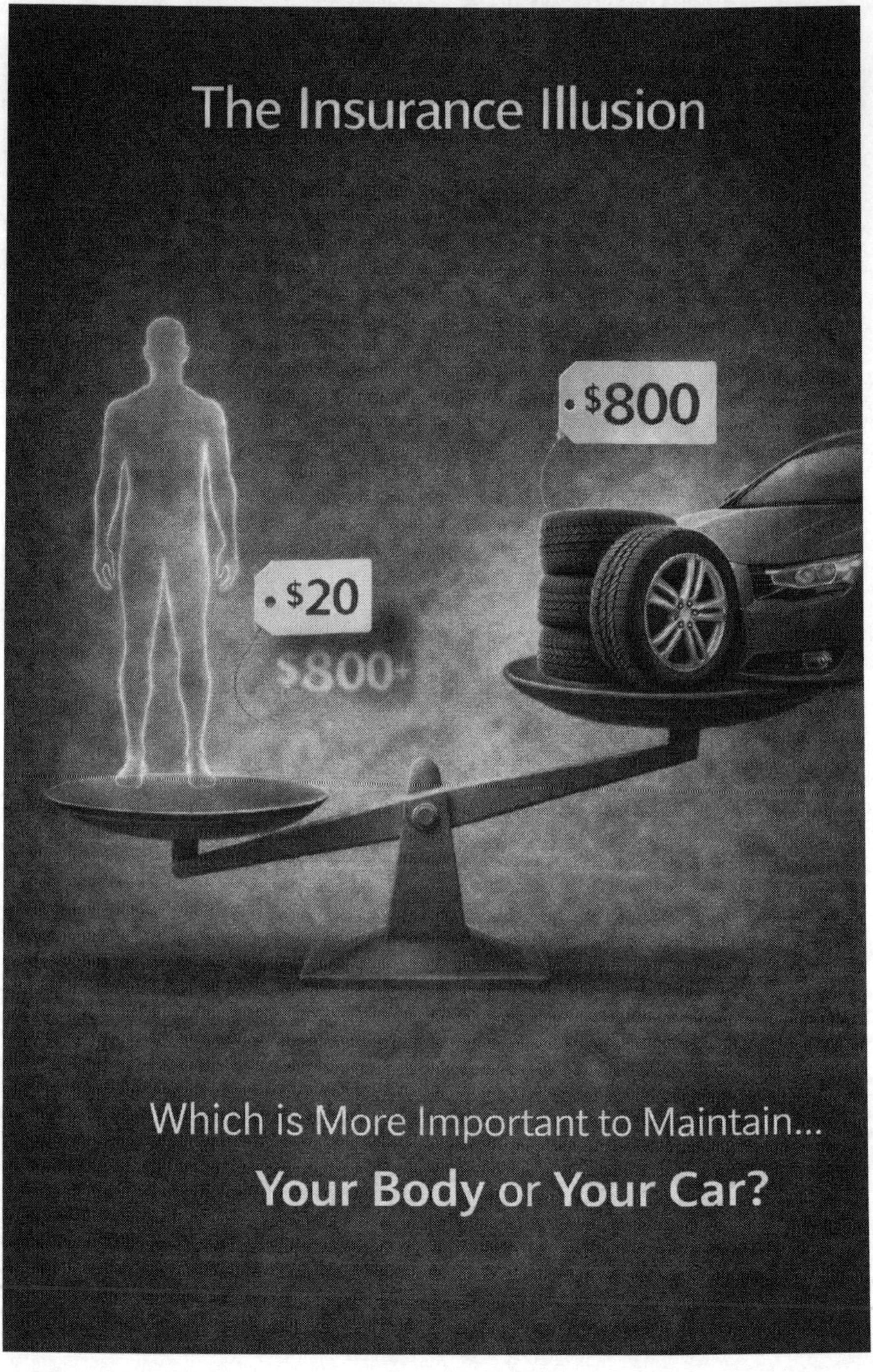
The Insurance Illusion
$800
$20
$800+
Which is More Important to Maintain...
Your Body or Your Car?

For some reason, they think health insurance should cover all costs. It doesn't.

I use the tire example with patients. Then I say "Your health, and your sexual health, are priceless. The investment in them is priceless."

You maintain your car because it needs to function correctly. You invest in tires because worn tires are dangerous.

Your body deserves at least the same consideration as your vehicle.

FINANCING AND PAYMENT OPTIONS

Payment Flexibility at Biltmore

Cash Payment Benefits

We offer Immediate payment discounts of 10-15% for upfront payment, thereby avoiding interest charges and financing costs. This simplifies the process and streamlines treatment scheduling. We also offer additional discounts for package deals.

Financing Programs

- CareCredit healthcare-specific financing with promotional rates
- In-house payment plans offering customized payment schedules
- Low-interest options with extended payment terms at reasonable rates
- No-credit-check plans provide options for those with credit challenges

Health Savings Accounts

- HSA eligibility, since some treatments may qualify for HSA funds
- FSA options allow for flexible spending account reimbursement
- Tax benefits are achieved using pre-tax dollars to reduce the effective cost
- Proper documentation is required for medical reimbursement

FINANCIAL PLANNING STRATEGIES

Budgeting for Treatment

Begin with a priority assessment to identify which treatments address your most pressing concerns first. Consider a phased approach that spreads treatments over time to make them more manageable financially. Seasonal planning can be strategic; timing treatments to coincide with bonus periods or tax refunds makes the investment easier. And if you have a supportive partner, partnership planning that involves sharing costs can make comprehensive treatment more accessible.

Cost-Benefit Analysis

A thorough cost-benefit analysis begins with a current spending audit, reviewing what you're already spending on health and wellness to see where sexual health treatment might fit. Consider the opportunity cost by comparing this investment to other major purchases or investments you're considering. Calculate the long-term savings you might realize from improved health and reduced medical needs down the road. And don't forget to assess the quality-of-life value —those non-monetary benefits that significantly impact your daily happiness and satisfaction.

The Marriage Economics

My practice saves marriages.

That's not hyperbole. Women who haven't initiated sex in years suddenly look forward to intimacy. That strengthens marriages in ways that ripple through every aspect of life.

And saving marriages saves everyone, except the attorney, money.

Consider the actual financial cost of a struggling marriage. Marriage counseling runs hundreds of dollars per session, often for months or years. Divorce proceedings can cost $15,000 to $50,000 or more. Separate households double living expenses.

A $20,000 investment in comprehensive sexual health treatment starts looking very different when you compare it to the alternative.

By definition, once someone becomes my patient, their marriage improves. The investment generates returns immediately and continues to compound.

INSURANCE AND REIMBURSEMENT CONSIDERATIONS

Coverage Limitations

Typically NOT Covered

- Cosmetic procedures for enhancement or aesthetic purposes
- Elective treatments for non-medically necessary interventions
- Experimental therapies, including newer treatments without established coverage
- Optimization treatments for performance enhancement

Potentially Covered

Insurance may potentially cover diagnosed medical conditions, including treatment of documented erectile dysfunction with a precise medical diagnosis. Hormone deficiency requiring replacement therapy for clinically low levels sometimes qualifies for coverage. Psychological counseling for therapy addressing sexual dysfunction may be reimbursable through your mental health benefits. Diagnostic testing, including laboratory work and clinical evaluations, often receives at least partial insurance coverage.

MAXIMIZING REIMBURSEMENT POTENTIAL

Documentation Requirements

- Medical necessity through clear documentation of medical need
- Failed conservative treatment showing evidence of trying standard approaches first
- Specialist referral with recommendations from primary care physicians
- Objective testing through laboratory or other diagnostic evidence

Reimbursement Strategies

- Flexible spending accounts using pre-tax dollars for qualified expenses
- Health savings accounts maximize HSA benefits for medical expenses
- Tax deductions, taking medical expense deductions when applicable
- Partial coverage, where some components may be covered even if others aren't

The Five-Year Divergence

I've now seen enough patients over enough years to observe clear patterns.

Patients who invest upfront are happier, healthier, and look and feel better for those five years.

Patients who decline during those years often wait.

The divergence is measurable. Weight gain. Deeper wrinkles. Increased spouse alienation. Pre-diabetes progression. Osteoporosis development. Soaring cardiovascular risk.

The medical costs of managing pre-diabetes alone dwarf the upfront investment in hormone optimization. Add in the costs of treating osteoporosis or recovering from a cardiac event, and the economics become crystal clear.

Prevention costs less than treatment. Always.

But there's a window. The earlier you invest, the better the returns. The longer you wait, the more expensive the eventual intervention becomes and the less effective it may be.

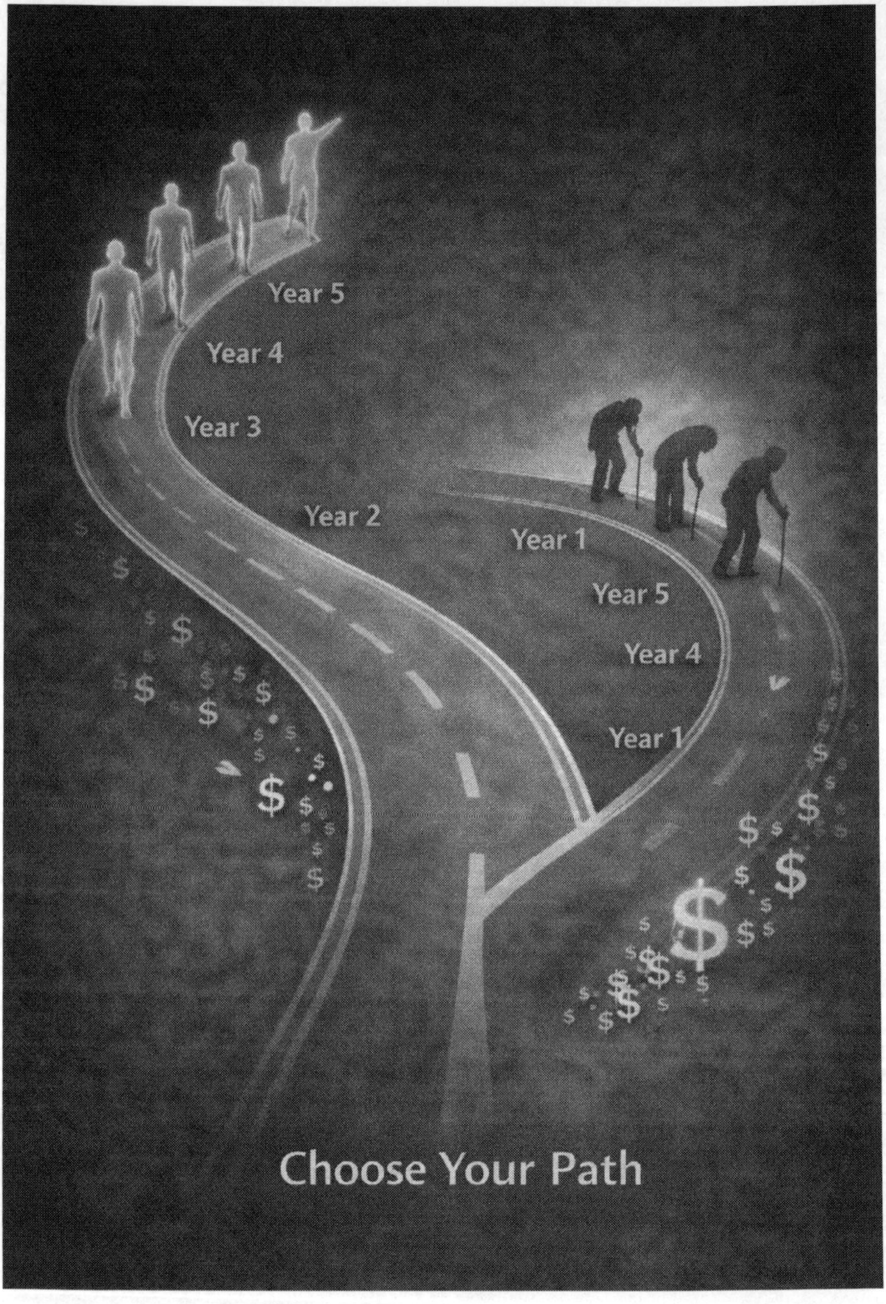
Year 5
Year 4
Year 3
Year 2
Year 1
Year 5
Year 4
Year 1
Choose Your Path

VALUE COMPARISON WITH ALTERNATIVE APPROACHES

Comparing Treatment Options

Prescription Medications

- Annual cost of $2,000-5,000 for ED medications
- Limitations in only addressing symptoms, not underlying causes
- Side effects, including potential cardiovascular and other risks
- Dependency creates an ongoing need without addressing the root problems
- Effectiveness that may decrease over time

Over-the-Counter Solutions

- Supplement costs of $1,000-3,000 annually for unproven products
- Device expenses of $200-1,000 for pumps, rings, and gadgets
- Effectiveness with limited scientific evidence for most products
- Safety concerns from unregulated products with unknown ingredients
- Disappointment from low success rates and wasted money

Surgical Interventions

- Penile implants costing $20,000-30,000 with irreversible changes
- Penile surgery at $15,000-25,000 with significant risks
- Recovery time of weeks to months of downtime
- Complications with a higher risk of serious adverse events
- Revision needs with potential need for future surgeries

THE BILTMORE RESTORATIVE MEDICINE ADVANTAGE

Comprehensive Value Proposition

- Expert care from a urologist with 30+ years of experience
- Advanced technology using the latest equipment and techniques
- Personalized approach with customized treatment plans for individual needs
- Ongoing support provides a long-term relationship and care
- Results-focused commitment to achieving your goals

Cost-Effectiveness

- Bundle pricing offering discounts for comprehensive treatment approaches
- Long-term relationships provide loyalty programs and continued care discounts
- No hidden fees with transparent pricing and all costs disclosed upfront
- Payment flexibility with multiple payment options to fit your budget

THE ECONOMICS OF DELAYED DECISION-MAKING COSTS OF WAITING

Progressive Decline

Sexual health problems typically worsen over time without intervention, and symptoms continue to become more pronounced. Hormonal decline accelerates with age and is compounded by lifestyle factors. The relationship strain that develops can lead to permanent damage if left unaddressed. And your self-confidence continues to erode as ongoing dysfunction affects your sense of capability and worth.

Missed Opportunities

Career advancement becomes hampered by the reduced confidence and energy that accompany sexual dysfunction. Relationship opportunities are lost due to the insecurity that comes with sexual health challenges. Your overall quality of life is diminished by ongoing health challenges that affect your daily functioning. And health complications from untreated hormonal imbalances can create cascading medical issues down the road.

Financial Impact

The financial impact compounds over time through the ongoing costs of ineffective treatments and medications that fail to address the root causes. Relationship counseling and potential divorce expenses can quickly exceed the cost of treatment. Lost earning potential from reduced performance and confidence affects your career trajectory. Increased healthcare costs resulting from declining overall health create a mounting financial burden.

THE COMPOUND INTEREST OF HEALTH INVESTMENT

Early Investment Benefits

Early investment offers significant advantages across multiple dimensions. Prevention allows you to address issues before they become severe and more difficult to treat. Efficiency improves because it's much easier to treat early-stage problems than advanced conditions. Success creates momentum, and initial improvements build your confidence and motivation to continue. Lifestyle integration becomes easier when you incorporate healthy changes gradually, rather than trying to reverse years of decline all at once.

Long-term Value Accumulation

The value accumulates over time through multiple channels. Health dividends manifest as improved health, reduced future medical costs, and prevention of expensive health crises. Relationship benefits compound as stronger relationships provide ongoing value that enriches your entire life. Career enhancement occurs naturally as increased confidence leads to professional success and advancement. And quality-of-life improvements enhance your enjoyment of activities and experiences year after year.

The Investment Framework

Sexual health optimization isn't a luxury; it's a necessity. It's a strategic investment with quantifiable returns across multiple life dimensions.

Relationship returns	Restored intimacy, reduced anxiety, strengthened partnership, and avoided divorce costs.
Health returns	Reduced cardiovascular risk, maintained bone density, better metabolic function, and avoided major medical expenses.
Quality of life returns	Increased confidence, improved appearance, renewed vitality, enhanced daily functioning.
Financial returns	Preserved marriage, avoided medical costs, maintained career performance, reduced therapy expenses.

These returns compound over time. Year-one benefits carry over into year two. Year-two improvements enable year-three advances.

Meanwhile, the alternative compounds are in the reverse order. Each year of delay makes the decline in the next year steeper.

MAKING THE FINANCIAL DECISION – INVESTMENT DECISION FRAMEWORK

Phase 1: Assessment and Prioritization

Phase 1 begins with a thorough assessment and prioritization process. Start with a current cost analysis to calculate what you're already spending on sexual health issues and ineffective solutions. Then, prioritize the treatments to determine which ones will address your most important concerns first. Assess your financial capacity by reviewing available resources and payment options. Finally, develop a timeline to create a realistic treatment schedule that aligns with your budget and goals.

Phase 2: Value-Based Decision Making

Phase 2 focuses on value-based decision-making that extends beyond price alone. Conduct a benefit analysis that compares potential outcomes to the investment required. Do an alternative comparison to evaluate all available treatment options side by side. Complete a risk assessment that considers both financial and medical risks of each approach. And engage in long-term planning that accounts for ongoing costs and maintenance needs, so there are no surprises down the road.

Phase 3: Implementation Strategy

Phase 3 is about creating your implementation strategy. Begin by selecting your payment method to choose the most suitable approach for your situation. Work on treatment sequencing to plan the order of treatments for maximum benefit. Build your support system to ensure you have adequate financial and emotional support throughout the process. Establish a monitoring plan to track both your financial investment and health outcomes as you progress.

COMMON FINANCIAL CONCERNS AND SOLUTIONS

"I Can't Afford It"

When patients say, "I can't afford it," I encourage them to conduct a reality check by comparing this investment to other discretionary spending in their lives. We offer payment plans that utilize financing to spread the costs over time, making treatment more affordable. Consider a priority adjustment, review what you're currently spending on ineffective solutions that could be redirected to treatments that actually work. We can implement a phased approach, starting with the most essential treatments first and building upon them.

"It's Too Expensive"

When confronted with "It's too expensive," I walk patients through a comprehensive value analysis. Calculate the cost per day or month over the benefit period; it's often less than their daily coffee budget. Consider comparing our treatments with alternatives such as surgery, medications, or devices; our treatments are usually less expensive and deliver better outcomes. Factor in quality considerations, including provider expertise, safety record, and actual results. And adopt a long-term perspective by considering the lifetime value versus the initial cost, prevention is always cheaper than treating advanced problems.

"What If It Doesn't Work?"

For those worried, "What if it doesn't work?", I address this concern by pointing to our track record. Review the published success rates for these treatments; they're backed by solid research and clinical evidence. Provider experience matters enormously, and you should always choose experienced, qualified providers with proven track records. Realistic expectations are crucial; we ensure you understand the likely outcomes before you begin. Follow-up care demonstrates our commitment; we verify our provider's dedication to your success through comprehensive ongoing support.

"Insurance Won't Cover It"

Utilizing an HSA/FSA to take advantage of tax-advantaged accounts may be an option. This typically requires medical necessity documentation, which can be obtained by working with the provider to document the medical need. Take advantage of tax savings for medical expense deductions when applicable.

MAXIMIZING YOUR INVESTMENT VALUE OPTIMIZING TREATMENT OUTCOMES

Pre-Treatment Optimization

Before treatment begins, focus on pre-treatment optimization to prepare your body and mind for success. Enhance your health status by optimizing your overall well-being through basic wellness practices. Address lifestyle factors —including diet, exercise, sleep, and stress management — to build the best foundation. Engage in expectation-setting to ensure you have a realistic understanding of the outcomes you can expect and when to expect them. Activate your support system by engaging with your partner and family so they understand the journey and can offer the support you need.

During Treatment

- Compliance by following all treatment protocols carefully
- Communication, maintaining an open dialogue with your provider
- Monitoring, tracking progress, and reporting any concerns
- Patience, allowing adequate time for treatments to work

Post-Treatment Maintenance

- Lifestyle continuation, maintaining healthy habits long-term
- Follow-up care, keeping all scheduled appointments
- Touch-up treatments and pursuing maintenance as recommended

The Real Question

When someone sits in my office wearing expensive jewelry and driving an expensive car, I don't judge their priorities.

But I do ask them to examine their calculation.

You've already demonstrated that you have the resources to invest in what you value. The question isn't whether you can afford sexual health optimization.

The question is whether you can afford not to.

What will the next five years cost if you don't invest? What will your marriage look like? What will your health markers show? What will your quality of life be?

And what will it cost to address those problems once they've compounded for five years?

I'm not ashamed of what comprehensive sexual health treatment costs. I'm proud of what it delivers.

High-quality care from highly trained, experienced providers produces life-changing results. The investment is justified by the returns it generates.

CONCLUSION: INVESTMENT IN YOUR BEST SELF

The decision to invest in sexual health treatment is ultimately a decision to invest in yourself, your relationships, and your future quality of life. While the financial commitment is significant, the men who proceed with comprehensive treatment consistently tell us it was one of the best decisions they've ever made.

At Biltmore Restorative Medicine & Aesthetics, we understand that this is a major financial and personal decision. We're committed to providing transparent pricing with no hidden fees or surprise costs, so you know exactly what to expect. Payment flexibility is a priority; we offer multiple options designed to fit your budget and make treatment accessible. Value maximization drives everything we do, ensuring you receive optimal results for your investment. And we believe in building long-term relationships that support your success well beyond the initial treatment phase.

Remember that the cost of inaction often exceeds the cost of treatment. Every day you wait is another day of diminished quality of life, relationship strain, and missed opportunities for improvement. The treatments we offer have helped thousands of men reclaim their vitality, confidence, and satisfaction with life.

Your sexual health is not a luxury; it's a fundamental component of your overall well-being and quality of life. When viewed in this context, the investment in comprehensive sexual health treatment becomes not just reasonable but essential for the man who wants to live his best life.

Your sexual health is priceless. But the cost of neglecting it is very, very quantifiable.

The math is straightforward. The choice is yours.

The question isn't whether you can afford to invest in your sexual health, it's whether you can afford not to.

References

Yeap BB, Alfonso H, Chubb SA, et al.
Are declining testosterone levels a major risk factor for ill-health in aging men?
Int J Impot Res. 2009;21(1)24-36. PMID 19037223
https//pubmed.ncbi.nlm.nih.gov/19037223/

Wu FC, Tajar A, Beynon JM, et al.
Testosterone and ill-health in aging men.
Eur J Endocrinol. 2009;160(6)1029-1039. PMID 19165223
https//pubmed.ncbi.nlm.nih.gov/19165223/

Corona G, Rastrelli G, Giagulli VA, et al.
Testosterone Therapy What We Have Learned From Trials.
J Sex Med. 2020;17(3)447-460.
PMID 31928918
https//pubmed.ncbi.nlm.nih.gov/31928918/

CHAPTER 9

Your Results Roadmap: What to Expect and When

The Sexual Health Timeline That Surprises Everyone

Men walk into my office expecting something entirely different.

They're used to injuries that take months to heal. Sports medicine timelines. Surgical recovery periods. They brace themselves for a long, slow climb back to vitality.

Then testosterone optimization hits them like a car going from zero to sixty.

One day, they're tired and listless. A few days later, they're energetic and full of vigor. The shift catches them off guard because it contradicts everything they thought they knew about medical treatment timelines.

But here's where it gets interesting.

That initial acceleration isn't the finish line. It's the starting gun.

Setting Realistic Expectations for Your Journey

After three decades of helping men restore their sexual vitality, I've learned that the most satisfied patients are those who understand precisely what to expect throughout their treatment journey. At Biltmore Restorative

Medicine & Aesthetics, informed patients make better decisions, comply more effectively with treatment protocols, and achieve better outcomes. This chapter provides a comprehensive roadmap of what to expect from each treatment, when to expect it, and how to maximize your results.

UNDERSTANDING THE TIMELINE OF SEXUAL HEALTH IMPROVEMENT

The Reality of Biological Change

Sexual health restoration is a biological process that takes time. Unlike a surgical procedure, where results are immediate, regenerative and optimization treatments work by stimulating your body's natural healing and restoration mechanisms. This biological reality means

- Results develop progressively over weeks to months
- Timeline varies based on age, health status, and treatment response
- Improvements often build upon each other over time
- The best results come to those who allow adequate time for biological changes

Factors Affecting Timeline

Several key factors influence how quickly you'll experience results from treatment. Younger patients often respond more quickly to treatments because their bodies retain greater regenerative capacity. Your overall baseline health plays a crucial role—if you're starting from a stronger foundation, you'll typically see faster improvement. Lifestyle factors, such as exercise, nutrition, and sleep quality, all significantly impact your response time and treatment outcomes. Treatment compliance is essential; following protocols precisely optimizes your results and accelerates progress. Finally, realistic expectations matter—understanding normal timelines reduces anxiety and helps you appreciate gradual improvements rather than becoming discouraged by unrealistic hopes for instant transformation.

The Zero to Sixty Phenomenon

Within days to a week of starting testosterone optimization, many patients feel something shift.

The effects reach a new baseline in about four to six weeks. This baseline sits significantly higher than where they started. Mental fog clears. Confidence rebuilds.

After six weeks, they're cruising on cruise control.

Mood improves. Foggy thinking clears. Relationships strengthen as things improve in the bedroom. They're not just functioning better. They're enjoying life in a way they'd forgotten was possible.

But optimal results? Those take longer if dose adjustments or timing intervals need fine-tuning.

This creates a strange paradox. Immediate effects that still require patience for optimization.

HORMONE OPTIMIZATION RESULTS TIMELINE TESTOSTERONE REPLACEMENT THERAPY PROGRESSION

Week 1-2: Initial Adaptation

Physical changes remain minimal, and visible changes are rare. Energy levels may show subtle improvement in some patients. Mood may fluctuate as the body adapts. Sleep patterns may change. Sexual function usually indicates no significant changes yet.

Week 3-4: Early Response

Energy levels show more noticeable improvement in vitality. Mood enhancement reduces irritability and increases motivation. Sleep quality shows better sleep patterns beginning to establish. Physical changes remain very subtle in muscle tone. Sexual interest may start with a slight increase in libido.

Week 6-8: Momentum Building

Energy shows significant improvement in daily energy and stamina. Mood brings notable enhancement in overall mood and outlook. Physical changes begin to show changes in body composition. Sexual function improves with morning erections and increased sexual thoughts. Cognitive function shows better mental clarity and focus.

Month 3: Substantial Improvement

Physical transformation becomes noticeable with increased muscle mass and reduced fat. Energy and vitality show a dramatic overall improvement. Sexual function significantly enhances in erectile quality and libido. Mood stability shows consistent improvement in emotional well-being. Sleep establishes a pattern of quality, restorative sleep.

Month 6: Optimal Benefits

Peak physical changes are typically associated with the most significant improvement in body composition. Sexual performance reaches optimal enhancement in all aspects of sexual function. The quality of life shows a dramatic improvement in overall life satisfaction. Relationship benefits enhance intimacy and communication. Confidence shows a significant boost in self-assurance and motivation.

Month 12 and Beyond: Maintenance Phase

Sustained benefits maintain improvements with continued treatment. Fine-tuning involves adjusting the dosage to achieve optimal long-term results. Preventive benefits protect against age-related decline. Health optimization continues to benefit cardiovascular and metabolic health.

TWO ROADS TO THE SAME DESTINATION

The delivery method you choose shapes your entire experience.

Injections accelerate rapidly and abruptly. Implants or pellets follow a slower but steadier journey with less fluctuation.

Think of it as choosing between a sports car and a luxury sedan. Both get you there. The ride may feel different.

Not all men experience the highs and lows of injections. But some do.

I lay out both options clearly. Some patients have already been on injections and want to continue. Others fear needles, so implants appeal to them immediately.

The investment remains the same regardless of whether you choose creams, injections, or implants. So, the decision comes down to biology and psychology.

How well can you handle an erratic journey versus waiting for a slower, more stable build?

I let patients decide. I also tell them they can switch methods if their initial choice doesn't align with their experience.

When the Spouse Becomes the Mirror

Sometimes patients don't see what's happening until someone else points it out.

A typical example: The man whose spouse tells him that two days after each injection, he's acting like a prick.

He's experiencing peak testosterone levels at day two. The surge creates irritability he can't see in himself.

I tell him we can cut his dose and inject more frequently. Or switch to implants for a smoother ride.

Road rage appears. Snapping at colleagues at work. These signs tell me a patient is riding the testosterone wave rather than maintaining steady optimization.

This whole phenomenon is rare. But it can happen.

The spouse-as-mirror moment reveals a crucial aspect of optimization. You're not just chasing numbers on a lab report. You're calibrating biology to match daily life.

The Happy Line

I think about hormone optimization in terms of curves.

All medications follow a pattern. They start low, reach a peak, then decline.

Injections create a rapid rise and fall. Implants produce a gradual rise and fall.

Somewhere along that decline sits what I call the "happy line." It's the level where patients feel optimized. Drop below it, and they notice.

For women, implants tend to drop below the happy line at three months. For men, it's closer to four months.

This isn't arbitrary. It's biology expressing itself through predictable patterns.

Understanding the happy line changes how patients think about their treatment. They're not waiting for some distant finish line. They're maintaining a level that keeps them cruising.

The Compound Effect

Testosterone optimization runs on its own track. P-Shot and acoustic wave therapy work in tandem.

But P-Shot and acoustic wave therapy? They interact.

Improvements in cellular function from combining these treatments occur over 3 months. To maximize benefit, you add the second round before that three-month improvement period ends.

Think of a freight train. It speeds up, then slows down.

Keeping it moving is far easier when it's still rolling. Let it stop altogether, and starting it again requires a massive amount of energy.

The treatments compound on themselves. 1+1 equals 5, not just 2.

A man reports improvements in erectile quality after one combination session. After his second session? He tells me he's Superman in bed.

That shift from "improvement" to "Superman" represents more than physical change. It's a psychological transformation.

Confidence returns. Performance anxiety dissolves. The bedroom becomes a source of connection rather than stress.

The Six-Month Realization

Around six months, something shifts in how patients talk about their treatment.

They stop focusing exclusively on sexual function. They start to notice how this journey has changed aspects of their life they didn't even know were connected.

The phrase I hear most often at the six-month mark?

"Damn, I should have started seeing Dr. Ibrahim years ago."

They're not just talking about the bedroom. They're talking about energy at work. Patience with family. Clarity in decision-making. Confidence in social situations.

The treatment becomes a lens that brings everything else into focus.

This realization doesn't happen at week four or even month three. It emerges after sufficient time has passed for the changes to become integrated into daily life.

The biological optimization creates space for psychological transformation. But that transformation needs time to unfold.

REAL PATIENT SUCCESS STORIES AND TIMELINES

Case Study: The Comprehensive Transformation

Patient Profile: Mark, 48-year-old executive with low testosterone, erectile dysfunction, and declining confidence.

Treatment Protocol

- **Month 1:** Hormone optimization initiation
- **Month 2:** P-Shot® treatment
- **Month 3:** Acoustic wave therapy series
- **Month 4:** Priapus Toxin® treatment
- **Ongoing:** Lifestyle optimization and maintenance

Results Timeline

- **Month 1:** "I started feeling more energy within a few weeks of starting testosterone therapy."
- **Month 2:** "The P-Shot® gave me hope that things could really improve."

- **Month 3:** "By the end of acoustic wave therapy, my erections were the best they'd been in years."
- **Month 4:** "The Priapus Toxin® was the icing on the cake - my confidence went through the roof."
- **Month 6:** "I feel like I'm 30 again. My wife and I couldn't be happier."
- **Year 1:** "This investment changed my life. I wish I had done it years ago."

The Timeline Nobody Warns You About

Here's what the journey actually looks like.

- **Days 1-7:** The acceleration begins, energy shifts. Mental clarity improves. You feel something happening.
- **Weeks 2-6:** You reach your new baseline. Mood stabilizes at a higher level—confidence returns. Physical changes become noticeable. Bedroom performance improves.
- **Months 3-4:** You're cruising. The happy line holds steady. Life feels manageable again. You're not fighting against your own biology anymore.
- **Month 6:** The realization hits. This isn't just about sexual health. It's about restoring vitality across every dimension of life.
- **Month 12 and beyond:** Maintenance becomes intuitive. You understand your body's signals. You know when levels drop below the happy line. You're not chasing optimization anymore. You're living it.

The timeline surprises patients because it contradicts itself. Immediate effects that require long-term commitment. Rapid acceleration that demands patience. Physical changes that unlock psychological transformation.

The Choice That Changes Everything

I don't push patients toward specific treatments or timelines.

I explain the biology. I share the patterns I've observed. I describe what other patients experience.

Then I let them choose.

Some men are ready to start immediately. They schedule consultations, optimize their health markers, and begin treatment within four weeks.

Others need more time. They spend months educating themselves, improving their baseline health, and planning their finances. That's a valid path too.

The treatment works when patients understand what they're committing to. Not just the financial investment or the time commitment. However, the psychological shift required to embrace gradual optimization while experiencing immediate effects is significant.

Sexual health restoration isn't a quick fix. It's a recalibration.

Your biology didn't decline overnight. Restoring it requires patience, even when the initial effects surprise you with their speed.

The men who succeed understand this paradox. They celebrate the zero-to-sixty acceleration while respecting the longer journey to optimization.

They trust the curve. They maintain their position above the happy line. They stack treatments before momentum dies.

And at six months, they look back and wish they'd started sooner.

YOUR NEXT STEPS

If You're Ready to Begin

Immediate Actions

- **Schedule Consultation:** Book a comprehensive evaluation with a qualified provider
- **Prepare Questions:** List concerns and objectives for discussion
- **Gather Information:** Compile medical history and current medications
- **Financial Planning:** Finalize payment strategy and budget
- **Support System:** Engage partner and family support for the journey

Preparation Timeline

- **Week 1:** Schedule consultation and gather medical records
- **Week 2:** Complete pre-treatment health optimization
- **Week 3:** Finalize treatment plan and financial arrangements
- **Week 4:** Begin treatment protocol and lifestyle modifications

IF YOU NEED MORE TIME

Continued Preparation	
Education	Continue learning about treatment options and outcomes
Health Optimization	Begin lifestyle improvements while considering treatment
Financial Planning	Develop a savings strategy for future treatment
Support Building	Work on relationship communication and support
Goal Clarification	Continue refining personal objectives and expectations

Decision Timeline	
3 Months	Complete health optimization and financial planning
6 Months	Reassess readiness and treatment options
12 Months	Final decision point with continued health decline consideration

CONCLUSION: YOUR JOURNEY TO TRANSFORMATION

Understanding what to expect and when is crucial for success with sexual health treatment. The journey requires patience, commitment, and realistic expectations, but the rewards can be life-changing. Men who follow comprehensive treatment protocols and maintain healthy lifestyles consistently achieve remarkable improvements in sexual function, confidence, and overall quality of life.

That's the timeline nobody warns you about. Immediate enough to shock you. Gradual enough to require commitment. Transformative enough to make you wonder why you waited.

The choice is yours. The biology is predictable. The outcome depends on whether you're willing to trust the process even when it contradicts your expectations.

Because sexual health restoration feels backward until you understand it's actually right on time.

At Biltmore Restorative Medicine & Aesthetics, we're committed to guiding you through every step of this journey. Our experience with thousands of patients has taught us that informed, prepared, and committed patients achieve the best outcomes. We provide the expertise, technology, and support you need to reclaim your vitality and confidence.

Your results roadmap is a journey of transformation that extends far beyond sexual health. It's about becoming the best version of yourself... confident, vital, and fully engaged in life. The men who complete this journey consistently tell us it was one of the best decisions they've ever made.

The question isn't whether these treatments work... the evidence is clear. The question is whether you're ready to begin your journey to renewed vitality and confidence. When you are, we're here to guide you every step of the way.

References

Lange D, Bocchini-Martins DA, Resende RB, et al.
Long-term outcomes after low-intensity extracorporeal shock wave therapy for erectile dysfunction 3 years of follow-up.
Int Braz J Urol. 2024;50(6)672-682.
PMID 39422490
https//pubmed.ncbi.nlm.nih.gov/39422490/

Alkandari MH, Touma N, Carrier S.
Erectile dysfunction Is platelet-rich plasma the new frontier for treatment?
Front Reprod Health. 2022;4944765.
https//pmc.ncbi.nlm.nih.gov/articles/PMC9580815/

Wang Y, Chen F, Ye L, et al.
Age-related testosterone decline mechanisms and intervention strategies.
Reprod Biol Endocrinol. 2024;22140.
https//pmc.ncbi.nlm.nih.gov/articles/PMC11562514/

CONCLUSION

Taking the First Step Toward Your Best Self

The Journey We've Shared

Throughout this comprehensive guide, we've explored the complex landscape of modern male sexual health, from the underlying causes of dysfunction to the cutting-edge treatments that can restore vitality and confidence. We've examined the science behind hormonal decline, the psychology of sexual performance, and the revolutionary non-surgical treatments that are transforming men's lives.

But knowledge alone isn't transformation. Real change requires action, commitment, and the courage to invest in yourself.

The Reality of Male Sexual Health Today

As we've discussed, sexual health challenges are affecting younger men at unprecedented rates. The combination of environmental toxins, chronic stress, sedentary lifestyles, and cultural pressures has created a perfect storm of sexual dysfunction. However, we've also entered an era of unprecedented treatment options, scientifically backed interventions that can address not just symptoms, but also root causes.

The treatments available today at Biltmore Restorative Medicine & Aesthetics represent decades of medical advancement

- Precision hormone optimization that goes far beyond simple testosterone replacement
- Regenerative medicine approaches like the P-Shot® harness your body's own healing power.
- Advanced enhancement procedures like Priapus Toxin® and RestoreMore that address both function and confidence
- Comprehensive acoustic wave therapy that can restore natural erectile function
- Integrated psychological support that addresses the mental components of sexual health

What Sets Our Approach Apart

After three decades in medicine, I've learned that lasting transformation requires more than just advanced treatments; it requires a partnership between patient and physician, built on trust, expertise, and shared commitment to your success.

Our Unique Advantages

Medical Expertise

- A urologist with 30+ years of specialized experience
- Duke University training and academic medical center background
- Continuous education and involvement in advancing the field
- Certification in the most advanced sexual health treatments available

Comprehensive Care

- Independent practice allowing for a personalized, non-franchise approach
- Integration of medical, psychological, and lifestyle interventions

- Long-term relationships are focused on your ongoing success
- Access to the latest technologies and treatment options

Patient-Centered Philosophy

- Realistic expectation setting and honest communication
- Respect for your individual goals and circumstances
- Flexible payment options and financing to make treatment accessible
- Ongoing support throughout your transformation journey

THE MEN WHO TRANSFORM THEIR LIVES

The most successful patients share specific characteristics that contribute to their outstanding outcomes.

Commitment to the Process

- Understanding that real change takes time and patience
- Willingness to follow treatment protocols precisely
- Investment in lifestyle optimization alongside medical treatment
- Openness to ongoing communication with the healthcare team

Realistic Expectations

- Clear understanding of achievable outcomes
- Patience with the timeline of biological change
- Appreciation for gradual improvement over instant gratification
- Recognition that sexual health is part of overall wellness

Partnership Approach

- Active participation in treatment planning and decision-making
- Honest communication about concerns, goals, and progress
- Commitment to follow-up care and maintenance
- Investment in the relationship with their healthcare provider

THE TRANSFORMATION POTENTIAL

The men who complete comprehensive sexual health optimization consistently experience improvements that extend far beyond the bedroom

Physical Transformation

- Increased energy and vitality throughout the day
- Improved muscle mass and reduced body fat
- Enhanced cardiovascular health and metabolic function
- Better sleep quality and recovery

Sexual Enhancement

- Dramatically improved erectile function and quality
- Increased sensitivity and pleasure
- Enhanced confidence and performance
- Renewed interest and desire

Psychological Benefits

- Significant boost in self-confidence and self-esteem
- Reduced anxiety and improved mood
- Better stress management and resilience
- Enhanced motivation and drive in all life areas

Relationship Improvements

- Renewed intimacy and connection with partners
- Improved communication and emotional closeness
- Enhanced relationship satisfaction for both partners
- Strengthened bonds and shared happiness

Professional and Social Benefits

- Increased confidence in professional settings
- Better performance and leadership capabilities
- Enhanced social interactions and networking
- Improved overall quality of life and life satisfaction

THE COST OF INACTION

While the investment in sexual health treatment is significant, the cost of inaction is often much higher.

Progressive Decline

- Sexual health problems typically worsen over time without intervention
- Hormonal decline accelerates with age and lifestyle factors
- Relationship strain can lead to permanent damage
- Self-confidence continues to erode with ongoing dysfunction

Missed Opportunities

- Career advancement hampered by reduced confidence and energy
- Relationship opportunities lost due to sexual insecurity
- Quality of life diminished by ongoing health challenges
- Health complications from untreated hormonal imbalances

Financial Impact

- Ongoing costs of ineffective treatments and medications
- Relationship counseling and potential divorce expenses
- Lost earning potential from reduced performance and confidence
- Increased healthcare costs from declining overall health

MAKING THE DECISION

The decision to pursue sexual health optimization is profoundly personal and shouldn't be rushed. However, it also shouldn't be delayed indefinitely while problems worsen and opportunities are lost.

Key Decision Factors

Personal Readiness

- Clear understanding of your goals and motivations
- Realistic expectations about outcomes and timeline
- Financial capacity for comprehensive treatment
- Support system, including partner and family

Professional Evaluation

- Comprehensive medical assessment by a qualified specialist
- Detailed discussion of treatment options and expectations
- Clear understanding of risks, benefits, and alternatives
- Confidence in your chosen healthcare provider

Timing Considerations

- Current life circumstances and stress levels
- Ability to commit time for treatment and recovery

- Financial planning and payment strategy
- Partner support and relationship readiness

Your Next Steps

If you've reached this point in the book, you're clearly serious about understanding your options and making an informed decision about your sexual health. The question now is what comes next?

IF YOU'RE READY TO BEGIN

Immediate Actions

- **Schedule a Consultation:** Contact Biltmore Restorative Medicine & Aesthetics for a comprehensive evaluation
- **Prepare for Your Visit:** Gather medical records, medication lists, and prepare your questions
- **Financial Planning:** Review payment options and financing to fit your budget
- **Support System:** Discuss your decision with your partner and enlist their support
- **Health Optimization:** Begin lifestyle improvements that will enhance treatment outcomes

Your First Consultation

- Comprehensive medical and sexual history review
- Physical examination and assessment
- Laboratory testing to evaluate hormone levels and overall health
- Detailed discussion of treatment options and recommendations
- Clear explanation of expected outcomes, timeline, and costs

IF YOU NEED MORE TIME

Continued Preparation

- **Education:** Continue researching and learning about your options
- **Health Improvement:** Begin optimizing diet, exercise, sleep, and stress management
- **Financial Planning:** Develop a savings strategy for future treatment
- **Relationship:** Work: Improve communication with your partner about sexual health
- **Goal Clarification:** Continue refining your personal objectives and expectations

Decision Timeline

- Set a reasonable timeline for making your decision (3-6 months)
- Continue monitoring how your current situation affects your quality of life
- Reassess your readiness and circumstances regularly
- Remember that early intervention is typically more effective than delayed treatment

THE BILTMORE RESTORATIVE MEDICINE PROMISE

When you choose Biltmore Restorative Medicine & Aesthetics, you're not just selecting a treatment provider... you're beginning a partnership focused on your long-term success and satisfaction.

Our Commitment to You

- **Expert Care:** Access to Dr. Ibrahim's three decades of specialized experience
- **Advanced Technology:** The latest equipment and most effective treatment protocols
- **Personalized Approach:** Customized treatment plans designed for your unique needs
- **Ongoing Support:** Long-term relationship and commitment to your continued success
- **Transparent Communication:** Honest discussion of options, expectations, and outcomes

Your Investment in Excellence

- Independent practice with physician-led care, not a franchise operation
- A urologist with academic medical center training
- Certified provider of the most advanced sexual health treatments
- Commitment to staying current with the latest advances in the field
- Focus on results, safety, and patient satisfaction

A Personal Message from Dr. Ibrahim

As I reflect on my thirty-year journey in medicine... from my days as a Duke University clinical professor to my current practice specializing in sexual health optimization... I'm constantly amazed by the transformation possible when men take control of their health and invest in their well-being.

The diagnosis of multiple sclerosis that ended my surgical career initially felt like a devastating setback. However, it led me to discover the incredible field of restorative medicine and hormone optimization. Through my own experience with these treatments, I learned firsthand their life-changing potential.

Every day, I witness men restore their vitality, confidence, and zest for life. I see marriages renewed, careers revitalized, and men discovering they can feel better in their fifties and sixties than they did in their thirties. These transformations remind me why I transitioned from surgery to sexual health optimization... because helping men feel like themselves again is just as meaningful as the life-saving surgeries I once performed.

Your sexual health isn't a luxury; it's a fundamental component of your overall wellbeing and quality of life. The treatments we offer aren't experimental or unproven; they're scientifically backed interventions with decades of research and thousands of success stories.

The men who achieve the best results are those who approach treatment as an investment in their future selves. They understand that fundamental transformation requires patience, commitment, and expert guidance. They're willing to invest not just financially, but emotionally and physically in the process of becoming their best selves.

YOUR INVITATION TO TRANSFORMATION

This book has provided you with comprehensive information about male sexual health optimization, but information alone doesn't create change. A fundamental transformation begins with a single step, the decision to prioritize your health and invest in your future.

Whether you're experiencing the early signs of sexual decline or have been struggling for years, effective solutions are available. The treatments we've discussed can help you.

Restore your energy and vitality.

- Restore sexual function and confidence.
- Strengthen your relationships and intimacy.
- Enhance your overall health and wellness.
- Feel like the best version of yourself.

The choice is yours. You can continue to accept decline as inevitable, spend money on ineffective solutions, and watch your quality of life diminish. Or you can take action, invest in proven treatments, and reclaim the vitality and confidence that define your best self.

The Time is Now

Every day you wait is another day of diminished vitality, missed opportunities, and compromised quality of life. The sooner you begin your journey toward optimal sexual health, the sooner you can start experiencing the benefits that extend to every area of your life.

Sexual health optimization isn't about vanity or superficial concerns. It's about restoring your masculine vitality and living life to its fullest. It's about being the husband, father, leader, and man you're meant to be.

Your transformation begins with a conversation.

Contact Biltmore Restorative Medicine & Aesthetics today to schedule your comprehensive consultation. Let's discuss your goals, evaluate your options, and develop a personalized plan to help you reclaim your prime.

We can't wait to help you feel like YOU again!

CONTACT INFORMATION

Biltmore Restorative Medicine & Aesthetics

1 Vanderbilt Park Dr. #230
Asheville, NC 28803
828.505.288

52249 Augusta St.
Greenville, SC 29605
864.695.1469

info@biltmorerestorative.com

BiltmoreRestorativeMedicine.com

Dr. George K. Ibrahim, MD, MBA

Urologist | Hormone Optimization Expert |Duke University-Trained | 30+ Years Experience | Certified P-Shot® Provider | Sexual Health Specialist

ABOUT THE AUTHOR

Dr. George K. Ibrahim is a urologist with 30+ years of experience and a fellowship-trained hormone optimization specialist who has dedicated his career to helping men and women restore their vitality and quality of life. As the founder of Biltmore Restorative Medicine & Aesthetics in Asheville, North Carolina, Dr. Ibrahim has become a leading authority in hormone replacement therapy, sexual wellness medicine, and regenerative treatments.

Before specializing in restorative medicine, Dr. Ibrahim practiced as a urologist-oncologist, where he spent decades helping men navigate the complex challenges of urological health and cancer treatment. His extensive surgical experience and deep understanding of men's health issues provided him with unique insights into the physical and emotional challenges men face as they age.

In 2013, following his own diagnosis with multiple sclerosis, Dr. Ibrahim made the difficult decision to retire from surgery. Rather than leave medicine entirely, he discovered a new calling helping people restore their health, vitality, and confidence through advanced hormone optimization and regenerative therapies. He immersed himself in specialized training, completing a fellowship with the American Academy of Anti-Aging Medicine to become one of the most highly trained physicians in hormone management.

Dr. Ibrahim's practice philosophy centers on a comprehensive, whole-person approach to wellness. He doesn't simply treat isolated symptoms or conditions—he evaluates each patient holistically, addressing the interconnected factors that affect health, performance, and quality of life. His unique background as a urologist gives him unparalleled expertise in men's sexual health, prostate health, and the intricate relationship between hormones and male vitality.

Beyond treating patients, Dr. Ibrahim is a passionate educator who speaks nationally on the dangers of andropause and menopause, and how hormone optimization represents the most natural and effective approach to reducing risks of cardiac disease, Alzheimer's, osteoporosis, and other age-related conditions. He has helped countless patients achieve remarkable improvements in energy, strength, mental clarity, and sexual function—transformations that inspired him to share his knowledge more broadly through *Restore Your Prime*.

Dr. Ibrahim's practice has grown to serve patients from across the country, with many traveling from major metropolitan areas like Charlotte and Atlanta to access his expertise. His commitment to excellence and patient-centered care has earned Biltmore Restorative Medicine a reputation as one of the premier sexual wellness and restorative medicine practices in the Southeast.

When he's not caring for patients or advancing the field of restorative medicine, Dr. Ibrahim treasures time with his three children—Taylor, Khoury, and George Philip—and his granddaughter, Lily Love. An avid sailor and outdoor enthusiast, he enjoys hiking, traveling, and cooking. He believes that living fully and pursuing passions at every age exemplifies the restored vitality he helps his patients achieve.

Dr. Ibrahim lives in Asheville, North Carolina, where he continues to transform lives one patient at a time, helping men restore their prime and reclaim the energy, confidence, and performance they deserve.

For more information, visit

BiltmoreRestorativeMedicine.com

AshevilleMaleHealth.com

AshevilleMaleEnhancement.com

HormoneTherapyAsheville.com

PShotAsheville.com

GreenvilleSCMaleHealth.com

GreenvilleSCMaleEnhancement.com

HormoneTherapyGreenvilleSC.com

PShotGreenvilleSC.com

Made in United States
Troutdale, OR
11/03/2026

56844381R00175